I0116434

COUPLE'S WORKBOOK

A Guide on Assisted Reproduction Technology

4th Edition

Samuel P. Marynick, MD, MS, FACP, FACE, HCLD/ELD, FCRB

Juan Correa-Pérez, PhD, HCLD/CC/ALD, CTBS, EMB

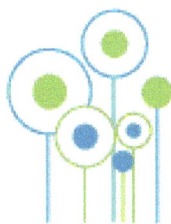

TEXAS CENTER FOR REPRODUCTIVE HEALTH

Copyright © 2016, Texas Center for Reproductive Health. All rights reserved. No part of this publication may be reproduced or transmitted in any form or by any means, electronic or mechanical, including photocopying, recording, or through an information storage and retrieval system, without permission in writing from the publisher.

Printed in the United States of America.

Texas Center for Reproductive Health and the associated logo are the trademarks of the Texas Center for Reproductive Health. The logo was designed by Ashley Popp, Susan Owen, and Sharon Marynick in 2010. All third-party marks are the property of their respective owners.

Texas Center for Reproductive Health is an active member of and certified by the Society for Assisted Reproductive Technology. Texas Center for Reproductive Health Laboratories are certified by the combined College of American Pathologists and American Society for Reproduction Medicine inspection process. The center laboratories participate in quality assurance and quality control monitoring through the College of American Pathologists and the American Association of Bioanalysts.

Address inquiries to the Medical Information Department, Texas Center for Reproductive Health, 3600 Gaston Avenue, Suite 504, Dallas, Texas 75246.

Previous editions: Copyrighted by the Texas Center for Reproductive Health:
    1st – 1990
    2nd – 1994
    3rd – 1997

ISBN: 978-0-9845237-2-6

"When you have exhausted all possibilities, remember you haven't."
—Thomas Edison (1847-1931)

"All excellent things are as difficult as they are rare."
—Benedict Spinoza (1632-1677)

"The reward of a thing well done is to have done it."
—Ralph Waldo Emerson (1803-1882)

"Despite our ability to manipulate and control human eggs and sperm using technology, conception remains and always will be, one of the deepest mysteries commanding our respect."
—Howard W. Jones, Jr., MD (1910-2015)

© 2016, Texas Center for Reproductive Health

Dedication

To our wives, Sharon and Nirma,
for their understanding and support
as we work to help our patients
realize their dreams.

Foreword

The first edition of this workbook was drafted in 1988 to help provide knowledge to couples involved in assisted reproduction procedures, in particular in vitro fertilization with embryo transfer (IVF/ET). At that point in time, there was no Internet material, little written material, and sparse information regarding these subjects.

As time has passed, the workbook has been refined; this edition is the third revision of the original document. Each revision has been undertaken with the goals of making current information available to patients and serving as a guide for patients as they participate in the IVF/ET process, which is often quite complex and challenging.

The authors' hope is that you will utilize this workbook to assist you in this challenging but potentially rewarding journey.

Samuel P. Marynick, MD, MS, FACP, FACE, HCLD/ELD, FCRB
Juan Correa-Pérez, PhD, HCLD/CC/ALD, CTBS, EMB
Dallas, Texas, January 2016

Table of Contents

List of Figures

Introduction

All around us the signs and symbols of fertility abound. Flowers bloom, newborns cry, and seasons change—simply and naturally. But for one in six couples who wish desperately for families, the procreative cycle stalls.

The Texas Center for Reproductive Health understands the powerful need to bear children that drives many couples with fertility problems. And we are sensitive to the frustration that mounts with each month if a pregnancy does not occur. Although we cannot guarantee a happy ending for everyone, we do offer to our patients state-of-the-art treatment technology that did not exist a few decades back.

The treatment programs available at the center intercede in the incredibly complex human reproductive process in order to help couples achieve a successful pregnancy. To accomplish this requires highly sophisticated assisted reproductive technology (ART) applied by clinical experts. But our clinical staff members are not the only active participants in this treatment. At the Texas Center for Reproductive Health, we consider you to be our partners.

The *Couple's Workbook* is our personal invitation inside the ART process. Through step-by-step descriptions of each phase of ART, from a couple's first meeting with a center professional through the treatment review, we explain what will happen, when, and why. We encourage you as a couple to participate in your treatment by studying the information provided here, by asking questions about any aspect of the treatment that is not clear to you, and by completing the medical record forms included in this workbook.

We hope the *Couple's Workbook*, written with assistance from fertility patients and professional counselors, will be your companion and guide during your evaluation and treatment.

WHAT'S INSIDE

❖ **Introductions to the treatment team.** To help couples get to know the center staff, this section offers a personal look at the backgrounds of the physician and embryologist who will be involved in your care.

❖ **Assisted reproductive technology.** The workbook starts with an explanation of the human reproductive cycle, followed by an overview of an ART cycle to illustrate how the treatment process "assists" in achieving pregnancy.

- ❖ **Evaluation.** The center physician will evaluate patient suitability for ART or other related therapies. Evaluations include a review of both the husband's and wife's medical records and, if applicable, further tests or physical examinations.

- ❖ **The treatment process.** A detailed explanation of each phase of the ART process addresses everything from the medications that start the cycle to fertilization to the pregnancy tests. Also included is a discussion of the option of cryopreservation if extra pre-embryos are available, as well as practical hints such as ways to handle multiple injections. The forms in this section may be completed by couples as their permanent record of the ART cycle. Each couple is given an individualized calendar to follow during their treatment at the Baylor Center for Reproductive Health.

- ❖ **Treatment review.** On completion of an ART treatment cycle at the Texas Center for Reproductive Health, each couple meets with a physician to discuss and evaluate the progression and results of the cycle.

- ❖ **Coping with stress.** Couples have to manage many complex and intense emotions during fertility treatment. This section features some techniques and recommended activities to keep your life steady while undergoing ART.

- ❖ **Financial considerations.** Money is usually a concern in fertility treatment. The latest information on insurance coverage, as well as suggestions for financing treatment, are discussed in this section. Fee schedules for the center are also available.

- ❖ **Appendices.** Appendices include charts showing center outcomes, a recommended reading list of books on infertility, a contact list with names and addresses of professional and support groups, fact sheets from ReproductiveFacts.org, and a glossary of terms relevant to the specialty of reproductive medicine.

HOW TO USE THE COUPLE'S WORKBOOK

Each couple undergoing ART receives a copy of the *Couple's Workbook* when beginning a treatment cycle. We encourage you as a couple to study the workbook together.

Read the detailed descriptions of each phase of the treatment cycle carefully. If you have questions, ask any of the center staff. Is the program what you expected? Have you made a decision about whether or not to use cryopreservation if you produce extra pre-embryos? Are you satisfied that ART is your best option?

When your treatment begins, the workbook becomes a constant companion as you record results of medication therapy, egg retrieval, or embryo transfer. Use the checklists and your program calendar to coordinate your visits. Complete the medical records forms at the end of each phase of the treatment as your reference.

The *Couple's Workbook* may also help you organize time. Examine the approximate timetable of the treatment cycle as shown on your program calendar and plan your schedule. Timing is extremely important in ART therapy, and once your treatment cycle begins, it may not be possible to make schedule adjustments. Practicing relaxation techniques before, during, and after ART treatment will help to relieve anxiety and make the program less stressful. Study and try the coping suggestions to see which approaches work for you. Plan your payments using the workbook's Financial Considerations section.

At the end of your cycle, whether successful or unsuccessful, review the notations made throughout the course of the treatment and prepare for a summary visit with a center professional to review the results and to discuss any appropriate next steps.

Your Treatment Team

Samuel P. Marynick, MD, MS, FACP, FACE, HCLD/ELD, FCRB

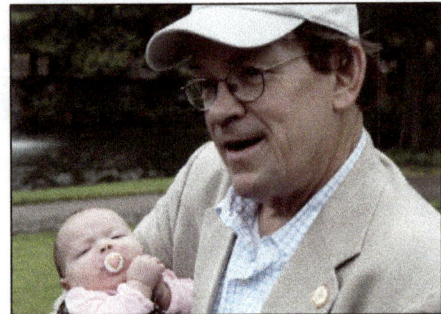

Dr. Marynick is both program and medical director for the Texas Center for Reproductive Health. He is board certified in internal medicine, endocrinology-metabolism, andrology, and embryology.

Dr. Marynick received his medical degree with Alpha Omega Alpha recognition from The University of Texas Southwestern Medical School in Dallas and completed his internship and residency in internal medicine at Parkland Memorial Hospital. From 1974 to 1977, he studied under world leaders in human reproductive medicine as a fellow in endocrinology at the Reproduction Research Branch in the National Institute of Child Health and Human Development at the National Institutes of Health in Bethesda, Maryland.

In 1977 he returned to Dallas and joined the staff of Baylor University Medical Center in the Internal Medicine Department's Division of Endocrinology. He began offering state-of-the-art reproductive medicine evaluation and treatment, including the use of Pergonal® for ovulation induction, which was not widely available at the time. In 1983, after attending a national symposium on in vitro fertilization with embryo transfer (IVF/ET) in Carmel, California, Dr. Marynick started developing the plan for an IVF and embryo transfer facility at Baylor University Medical Center.

Dr. Marynick opened his private practice in 1986, specializing in endocrinology and reproductive medicine. He has conducted both basic and clinical research in general and reproductive endocrinology, and the results of his studies have appeared in publications such as *The New England Journal of Medicine, The Journal of Clinical Investigation, The Journal of Clinical Endocrinology & Metabolism, Endocrinology, Fertility and Sterility,* and *The Annals of Internal Medicine.*

Dr. Marynick's professional interests extend beyond his own medical practice. Over the years, he has worked to train medical students, interns, residents, practicing physicians, and patients.

Having training and experience in both clinical and laboratory disciplines, Dr. Marynick served as the medical director and director of laboratories at the Baylor Center for Reproductive Health, Baylor University Medical Center, Dallas, Texas, from 1988 to 2001. During his tenure in that capacity, he was also the director of the Clinical Research

Program at the Baylor Research Institute of the Baylor Health Care System. From 2001 to 2005 he was the program director for the Baylor Center for Reproductive Health. He has the current distinction of being the program director and medical director of the Texas Center for Reproductive Health in Dallas, Texas.

Dr. Marynick is a Fellow of the American College of Physicians; a Fellow of the American College of Endocrinology; and a member of the American Association of Clinical Endocrinologists, the Endocrine Society, the American Society of Reproductive Medicine (serving on its Sessions Management Committee), the Reproductive Immunology Special Interest Group, the Society of Reproductive Endocrinology and Infertility, the American Society for Reproductive Immunology, the European Society of Human Reproduction and Embryology, the Reproduction Biology Professional Group, the American Association of Bioanalysts, the American College of Endocrinology, the College of Reproductive Biology, the Pituitary Network Association, the Thyroid Foundation of America, the Society for the Study of Male Reproduction and Urology, the American College of Physicians, the Texas Medical Association, the Dallas County Medical Society, and the Dallas Academy of Internal Medicine. He is also an attending physician at Baylor University Medical Center and has been a clinical associate professor in internal medicine (endocrinology/metabolism) at The University of Texas Southwestern Medical School since 1977.

Dr. Marynick has received numerous accolades and distinctions. In 1987, he was named an outstanding teacher and attending physician in internal medicine by Baylor University Medical Center at Dallas. He first made the distinguished list of "Top Doctors" by *D Magazine* in 1992 and has been named with this recognition consecutively since 2001. *Texas Monthly* magazine has included Dr. Marynick on its esteemed "Top Doctors in Texas in Reproductive Endocrinology and Endocrinology" list every year since 2004.

Dr. Marynick's certifications include the following: 1972, Texas State Board of Medical Examiners; 1973, National Board of Medical Examiners, Diplomate; 1975, American Board of Internal Medicine, Diplomate; 1975, Maryland Board of Medical Examiners; 1976, National Institutes of Health, Certificate of Training, Radioactive Materials; 1977, American Board of Internal Medicine, Diplomate in Endocrinology and Metabolism; 1994, American Board of Bioanalysis, Andrology; 1994, American Board of Bioanalysis, Embryology; 1994, American Board of Bioanalysis, Certified High Complexity Laboratory Director.

An active academic, board, and committee member and a highly requested speaker, Dr. Marynick has had the honor of authoring and coauthoring 55 publications.

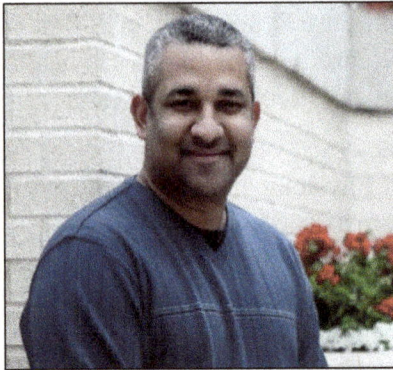

Juan Correa-Pérez, PhD, HCLD/CC/ALD, CTBS, EMB

An outstanding expert in the field of reproductive science, Dr. Correa-Pérez has a particular interest and expertise in male-factor infertility with an impressive resume of research.

Dr. Correa-Pérez is highly skilled in assisted hatching, retrieval of sperm from epididymal/testicular tissue, intracytoplasmic sperm injection, egg/embryo biopsy for preimplantation genetic screening or diagnosis, all aspects of andrology and embryology, sperm and embryo cryopreservation (freezing), and the treatment of severe male-factor infertility. He has a long and successful history of achieving impressive IVF success rates.

A dedicated patient advocate, Dr. Correa-Pérez is committed to excellence in patient care. He particularly enjoys educating patients about the IVF process to ensure their level of comfort, especially in regard to their own personal treatment or medical circumstances.

Dr. Correa-Pérez holds High-Complexity Clinical Laboratory Director and Clinical Consultant certifications granted through the American Board of Bioanalysis. He is also certified as a Tissue Banking Specialist by the American Board of Tissue Banking and as an Embryologist by the American College of Embryology. Extremely active in the professional community, he has served as a medical school faculty member, as well as an editorial board member for *The Scientific World Journal—Urology, The Open Andrology Journal,* and *Advances in Sexual Medicine Journal.* He is an ad hoc member of the editorial staff of *Fertility and Sterility* (a leading medical journal in the field of reproductive medicine) and a reviewer for several other outstanding journals in the field, including the *Journal of Andrology, Journal of Assisted Reproduction and Genetics, Asian Journal of Andrology, Urotoday International Journal,* and *Journal of Men's Health.* Dr. Correa-Pérez underwent formal training in 2006 at the Reproductive Genetics Institute in Chicago, Illinois, to perform advanced techniques in embryo biopsy for preimplantation genetic diagnosis. In 2009, he was invited to become a member of the National Registry of Volunteer Reviewers at the National Institutes of Health Center for Scientific Review.

As a researcher and scientist in reproductive physiology, andrology, and embryology, he is extensively published and has appeared in television, radio, newspaper, and magazine interviews on various infertility topics. He is a frequent invited lecturer in the related fields of obstetrics/gynecology and urology. He also enjoys speaking at support groups and other public forums.

Fluent in Spanish, Dr. Correa-Pérez assists with translation for our Spanish-speaking patients to facilitate their treatment and help them feel at ease.

Dr. Correa-Pérez received his bachelor's degree in animal sciences from the University of Puerto Rico, Mayaguez. He then completed a master's degree and PhD in reproductive physiology–andrology, with a statistics minor, from the University of

Kentucky. Afterwards, he was a postdoctoral fellow in reproductive physiology–andrology/medicinal chemistry and pharmacology at the University of Kentucky.

He is an active member of the following societies:

- American Society for Reproductive Medicine
- American College of Embryology
- American Society of Andrology
- International Society of Andrology
- Society for the Study of Male Reproduction
- Society for Male Reproduction and Urology
- American Association of Bioanalysts
- College of Reproductive Biology
- American Association of Tissue Banks
- Society for the Study of Reproduction
- Sigma Xi, The Scientific Research Society

Assisted Reproductive Technology

Couples who have not conceived after 1 year of unprotected intercourse have a fertility problem. More than 3.3 million couples suffer from such problems in the United States. The good news is that many of them can be treated with conventional therapy using medications or surgery. You are among the 500,000 couples, or about the 15% to 20% who may benefit from assisted reproductive technology (ART).

More than 35 years ago, the birth of Louise Brown, the world's first baby to be conceived by in vitro fertilization (IVF), brought new hope to childless couples. Today hundreds of thousands of babies have been born as a result of IVF, a term that literally means fertilized in glass.

What has transpired in the last few decades is miraculous. By manipulating the body's own natural cycle with fertility medications, specialists can produce and retrieve eggs, fertilize them outside the body, and return the fertilized eggs to the uterus, thus circumventing many obstacles to conception.

Approximately 25% of couples undergoing IVF give birth to a baby, according to the 1999 Society of Assisted Reproductive Technology report. In 1999, 86,822 cycles of IVF were performed nationwide, resulting in 30,285 babies. Each year success rates related to delivery of a baby improve as more is learned about the reproductive process. (Current success rates for **all** clinics can be found at www.sart.org and www.cdc.gov; outcomes for this center are shown in Appendix A.)

Although ART began as a solution for women with blocked tubes, it has become an accepted treatment for unexplained infertility, endometriosis (a disease where tissue that normally lines the uterus grows in the pelvic cavity outside of the uterus), and selected cases of immune system disorders, as well as male infertility.

THE HUMAN REPRODUCTIVE SYSTEM

The process of human reproduction is at once simple and complex, a marvel of precision orchestration and random chance. To understand why ART works, you need to know about the normal processes of ovulation, sperm production, and conception.

The Woman

A woman's reproductive organs are located completely inside her body (Figure 1). The female ovaries have two important functions: releasing one mature egg each menstrual cycle and producing the hormones estrogen and progesterone. (Refer to the next section,

"Unassisted Cycle," on page 11 for a more detailed description of the female reproductive cycle.)

The fallopian tubes are attached to the uterus by thin connective ligaments. Each tube is about 4 inches long with flower-like fimbria at the end closest to the ovary. The fimbria sweep the ovaries as they are releasing eggs and guide the eggs into the fallopian tubes. Inside the tubes, secretions released by glands in the tube smooth the way for eggs during their journey. Hair-like cilia that line the inner surface of the tubes create a wave-like motion that propels the eggs toward the uterus. The uterus, or womb, is pear shaped and pear sized, remarkably elastic, and muscular. During pregnancy, the uterus stretches from its usually compact size to accommodate a growing fetus.

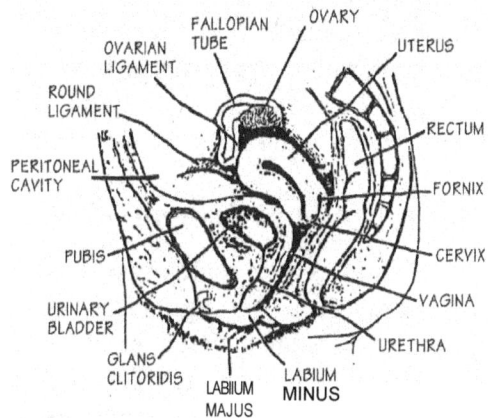

Figure 1. The female reproductive system.

The cervix is both the inhibitor and the facilitator of conception. Glands in the cervix secrete mucus throughout the menstrual cycle. This mucus varies in consistency to either encourage or discourage sperm from traveling further into the reproductive tract. The mucus at mid-cycle, during ovulation, is most conducive to sperm movement into the uterus. The cervix is a structure that guards the entrance of the uterus, or womb, where a fertilized egg would grow.

The vagina, about 3 to 5 inches in length, connects the uterus with the outside world.

The Man

A man's reproductive organs (Figure 2) are located outside as well as inside the body. The scrotum contains testes, blood vessels, nerves, and the vas deferens, which transports sperm from the testes to the urethra, a tube that runs through the penis. The scrotum's location behind the penis keeps the testes away from the body to maintain the lower temperature necessary for sperm production. The testes, hypothalamus, and pituitary gland orchestrate the continuous process of sperm generation called spermatogenesis. The hypothalamus stimulates the pituitary gland to produce follicle-stimulating hormone and luteinizing hormone. In the male, these hormones stimulate the testes to produce testosterone and

Figure 2. The male reproductive system.

sperm. Sperm mature in a complex tangle of tubes, or canals, in the testes over a 3-month period. After final development, it takes an additional 10 to 14 days of maturation in the ducts of the testes for sperm to be capable of natural egg fertilization.

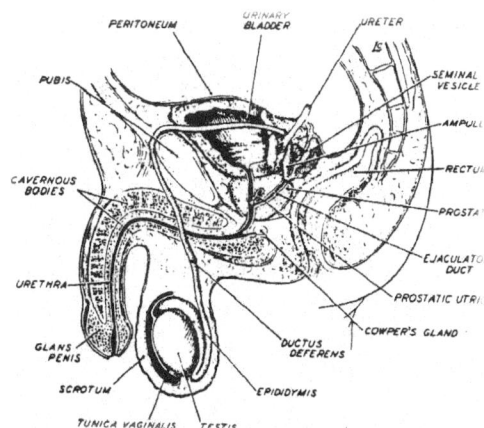

When the man becomes sexually excited, seminal fluid or semen (containing sperm, prostate secretions, and seminal vesicle secretions) moves from the duct system through the urethra and is expelled, or ejaculated, into the woman's vagina. Upon ejaculation, the substances that form the semen combine to coagulate, then reliquify within about 30 minutes. Sperm actively swim in seminal fluid once this fluid has reliquified. Failure of the semen to reliquify may diminish fertility by preventing the sperm from moving freely into the cervical mucus.

Conception and Pregnancy

Minutes after male orgasm, sperm begin their very long journey from the vagina through the uterus to the fallopian tubes. Their first obstacle is cervical mucus. Even with accommodating mid-cycle mucus, only a small fraction of the sperm in an ejaculation will survive this migration through the cervical mucus into the uterus.

For those sperm that do pass into the uterus, uterine contraction and their own swimming ability propel them at the speed of about 1 inch every 5 minutes to the top of the uterus. There the sperm enter the fallopian tubes. Some sperm initially remain in the fallopian tubes and may migrate out the fimbria and into the pelvis at a later time. Others swim out through the fimbria of the tube searching for an egg.

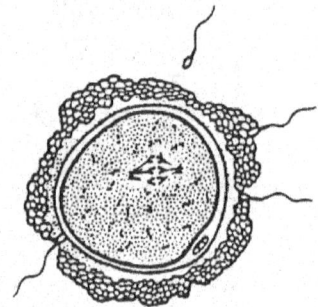

Figure 3. Schematic of sperm arriving at egg to begin fertilization.

Sperm undergo a process called capacitation during their journey through the female reproductive tract. During capacitation, the sperm's protective cap changes and releases enzymes that help the sperm penetrate the egg's protective cells and membrane.

Fertilization occurs when a sperm penetrates an egg and its chromosomes blend with those of the egg. Once a sperm penetrates an egg, a change occurs in the egg's protective membrane which prevents other sperm from entering the egg (Figure 3).

The zygote, as the fertilized egg is now known, divides repeatedly over the next few days as it moves down the fallopian tube. When it reaches the uterus, the zygote now has about 32 to 64 cells. If it successfully implants, a placenta starts to grow and cellular differentiation begins. Cellular differentiation is the process by which cells divide and give rise to new cells, some with specialized functions that are the beginning of the various body systems (i.e., neurological, circulatory, digestive).

Unlike men whose creation of reproductive cells is continuous, women undergo monthly cycles triggered by similar hormonal processes. Ideally a woman's reproductive cycle repeats itself every 26 to 34 days (28 days average) beginning when she enters puberty and ending with menopause. The teens and 20s are a woman's most fertile period, with a 20% to 25% chance of pregnancy per cycle (assuming unprotected intercourse). Age affects fertility, decreasing the chance of pregnancy to 8% per cycle in the late 30s and 40s. When menstruation begins, women have about 400,000 eggs. A woman typically ovulates a total of about 400 eggs in her life. Between the ages of 45 and 55, women have a cessation of fertility as the ovaries begin to fail. However, the ovaries continue to secrete some hormones at low levels for the remainder of the woman's life.

Each menstrual cycle has three distinct hormonal phases: **follicular, ovulatory, and luteal**. Figure 4 shows the interaction of hormones in the cycle.

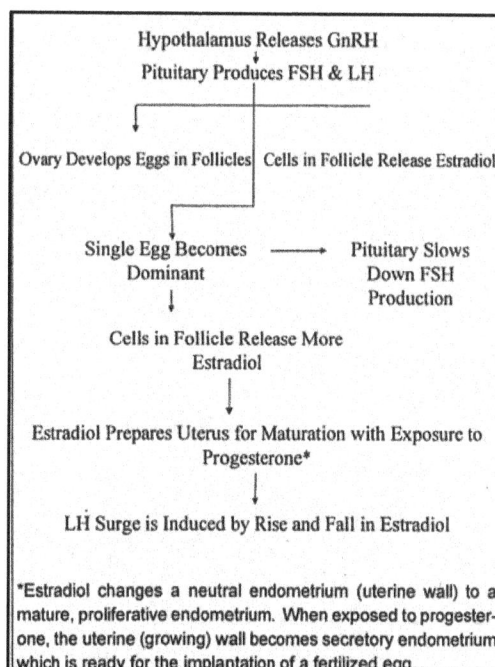

Figure 4. Interaction of hormones in the female menstrual cycle.

Follicular Phase

In the first half of a menstrual cycle, the hypothalamus releases gonadotropin-releasing hormone, which, in turn, signals the pituitary gland to produce follicle-stimulating hormone (FSH) and luteinizing hormone (LH) (Figure 5). In response to the FSH in the bloodstream, eggs begin to develop within each ovary, and the cells surrounding the egg release estradiol, the main hormone of the follicular phase. On about day 6 or 7, a single follicle containing a developing egg becomes dominant. An increased level of estrogen, produced by FSH stimulating the ovary, signals the pituitary gland to slow down the production of FSH, which causes other follicles to recede. At the same time, estradiol prepares the uterus for the luteal phase of the cycle by thickening the endometrial lining. When blood levels of estrogen peak and then drop (the result of complex interactions of FSH with the developing follicle), the stage has been set for the pituitary LH surge, which completes the maturation of the developing follicle.

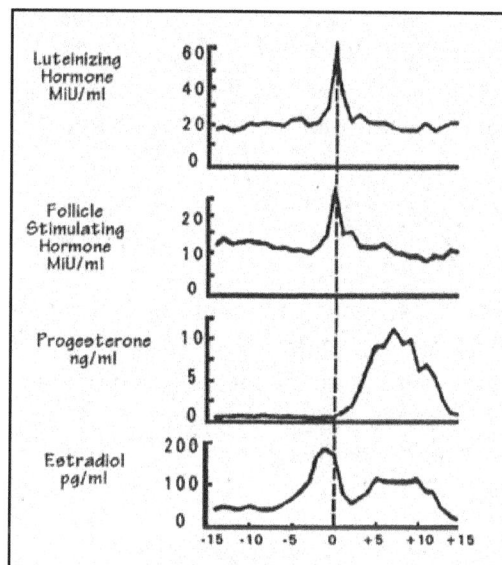

Figure 5. Follicular phase of the female menstrual cycle.

Ovulatory Phase

About **24 hours** after a natural LH surge, the wall of the follicle ruptures, releasing a mature egg. The egg is swept into the fallopian tubes by the fingers of the fimbria. There, if it is penetrated by a sperm and fertilized, it becomes a pre-embryo. This process typically takes place within 12 hours of ovulation, but can occur up to 24 hours after ovulation. The fertilized egg divides as it moves through the fallopian tube over the next 3 days and implants in the uterine wall (secretory endometrium) 6 days following fertilization.

Luteal Phase

Following ovulation, the ruptured follicle undergoes a transformation. Responding to the LH surge, cells in the follicle luteinize, which gives the follicle a yellow cast. It is now known as a corpus luteum, or "yellow body" in Latin. The job of the corpus luteum is to release progesterone and estrogen during the last half of the menstrual cycle. **A successful early pregnancy depends on adequate production of these hormones.**

If pregnancy occurs, human chorionic gonadotropin (hCG) appears in the bloodstream approximately 8 days after ovulation and stimulates the corpus luteum to continue producing progesterone well into the second trimester of the pregnancy. As the corpus luteum of pregnancy atrophies, the placenta takes over production of progesterone. If no pregnancy occurs, the lack of hCG in the blood allows the corpus luteum to discontinue production of progesterone and estrogen and the corpus luteum atrophies. The endometrium in the uterus, responding to lowered levels of progesterone, sheds the outer portion, and a menstrual flow begins.

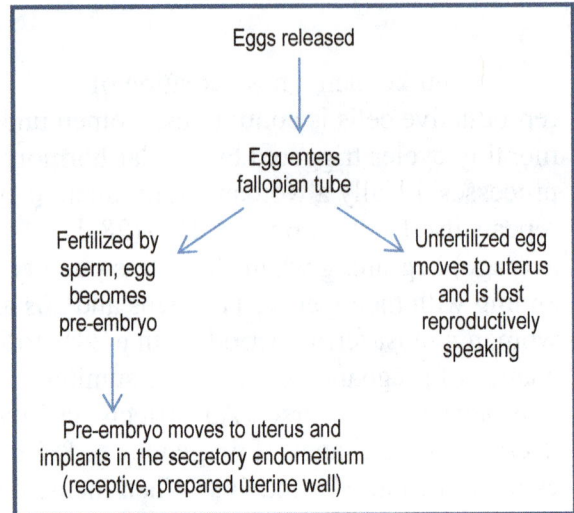

Figure 6. Ovulatory phase of the female menstrual cycle.

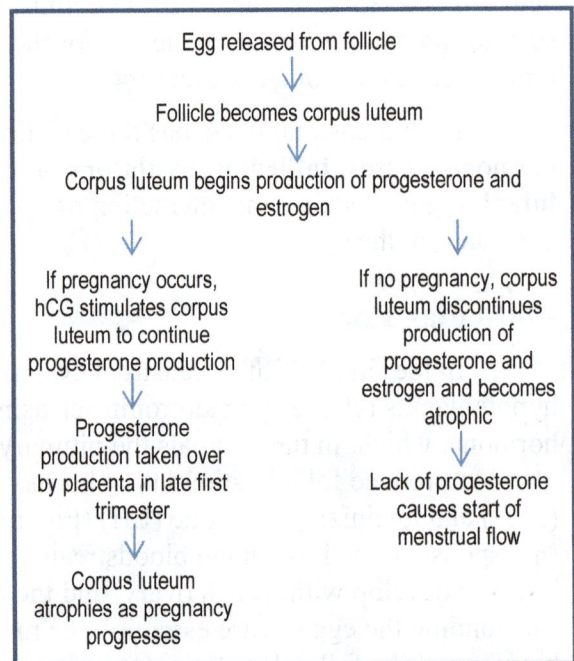

Figure 7. Luteal phase of the female menstrual cycle.

ASSISTED CYCLE

This is how an assisted reproductive technology (ART) cycle progresses at the Texas Center for Reproductive Health.

Luteal Phase

The ART cycle begins 3 weeks into a cycle of the oral contraceptive pill or in the luteal phase of a natural cycle, about 7 days after ovulation (21 to 23 days into the wife's cycle) with injections of Lupron. Lupron is a gonadotropin-releasing hormone agonist that stops the pituitary gland from releasing follicle-stimulating hormone (FSH) and luteinizing hormone (LH). By preventing the pituitary gland from releasing these two hormones, physicians can better control the development and maturation of follicles.

Follicular Phase

Without the stimulation from FSH and LH, the ovaries remain dormant. On day 2 or 3 of the assisted cycle, estradiol levels are measured and a sonogram performed to make sure no cysts over 15 millimeters exist on the ovaries. FSH, which is available under several brand names, is given to stimulate the ovaries to produce follicles. The initial dosage of FSH is designed to produce multiple follicles with mature eggs. If more than three ampules of medication are needed in any day of follicular stimulation, the ampules of medication are divided, with part being given in the morning and part in the evening.

Starting on about day 6 of FSH stimulation, women receive more frequent ultrasound examinations to measure follicular growth and maturation, as well as blood tests to check estradiol levels. Estradiol is an indirect measurement of follicular development. These tests identify when retrieval should be scheduled. Toward the completion of follicular stimulation, a small amount of LH is generally given in the form of the medication human menopausal gonadotropin, or hMG (for which there are several brand names). When estradiol levels and follicle size are adequate, one dose of human chorionic gonadotropin (hCG) is given. This matures the follicles so they are ready for egg retrieval.

Egg Retrieval

Egg retrieval is scheduled 34 to 35 hours after the dose of hCG is administered. Eggs are retrieved by vaginal sonogram. Eggs retrieved for in vitro fertilization are fertilized in vitro (in glass) in the center's embryology laboratory. Approximately 72 to 120 hours later, if fertilization has occurred, pre-embryos are returned to the wife's uterus.

In the ZIFT procedure, the retrieved eggs are combined with the husband's sperm, fertilization is confirmed, and the fertilized eggs, or zygotes, are placed in the wife's fallopian tubes approximately 24 hours after retrieval. We no longer perform this procedure at the Texas Center for Reproductive Health.

With GIFT therapy, eggs are retrieved and combined with the husband's sperm in the wife's fallopian tubes, all in one procedure. We no longer perform this procedure at the Texas Center for Reproductive Health.

After Egg Retrieval

Depending on the amount of estrogen the ovaries are releasing, an injection of hCG is generally given in the luteal phase of the cycle to stimulate the corpus luteum to produce progesterone and estrogen. Progesterone production allows the uterus to prepare for pregnancy. Supplemental progesterone is given by injection following egg retrieval daily to ensure that the uterus gets adequate hormone stimulation to change the endometrium or lining of the uterus to allow the uterus to implant a fertilized embryo, resulting in pregnancy.

Figure 8 compares the phases in an unassisted cycle and an ART cycle.

Figure 8. Unassisted cycle vs. IVF/ET cycle

Unassisted Cycle	Assisted Cycle
	Luteal Phase: 3 weeks into an oral contraceptive pill cycle or 7 days after ovulation, Lupron injections are given to suppress the pituitary's production of FSH and LH.
Follicular Phase: Ovaries respond to FSH and LH hormones released by the pituitary gland. Follicles containing eggs begin to develop. One follicle becomes dominant, and production of estradiol peaks.	*Follicular Phase:* On day 2 or 3 of the menstrual cycle during Lupron treatment, baseline estradiol measurements and sonograms are performed. FSH shots begin on day 3 to stimulate production of multiple follicles. Thirty-four to thirty-five hours before egg retrieval (about day 9 to 12 of FSH), hCG is given to trigger follicular maturation.
Ovulatory Phase: An LH surge causes the dominant follicle to rupture, releasing an egg. The egg moves into the fallopian tube to be potentially fertilized.	*Egg Retrieval:* Eggs are retrieved from multiple follicles by aspiration. An injection of progesterone is given. Eggs are fertilized in an embryology lab and are returned to the patient 72 to 120 hours later.
Luteal Phase: After releasing the egg, the follicle develops into the corpus luteum. Progesterone and some estrogen produced by the corpus luteum mature the uterine lining. If pregnancy occurs, the corpus luteum supports the developing pregnancy for several weeks. If no pregnancy develops, menstruation begins.	*Post Egg Retrieval:* Patient receives injections of progesterone following egg retrieval to develop the uterine lining. On day 4 following egg retrieval, an hCG shot may be given. Pregnancy tests are given on day 14 and, if positive, are repeated on day 16 after egg retrieval.

A pregnancy test is conducted at day 14 after the egg retrieval has taken place. If the test is positive, it is repeated at day 16. The first test identifies the earliest indication of pregnancy. The second test checks to see if the level of hCG has increased, confirming the presence of a developing placenta. If we see a positive hCG value that is rapidly increasing, this tells us a placenta is starting to grow to support the pregnancy. If the second test is positive and increasing, we can make some comment about how the pregnancy appears to be progressing.

Estrogen is frequently used by patients following egg retrieval to allow for adequate estrogen levels during pregnancy establishment and early pregnancy. Progesterone is given for several weeks to support the developing pregnancy. If pregnancy has not occurred, supportive medications will be stopped. In some cases hCG will be measurable but the levels will not be compatible with a viable ongoing pregnancy. Such a situation is referred to as a "biochemical pregnancy."

Evaluation

"I began my infertility workup with mixed feelings. It was a frightening, uncertain time. I couldn't get pregnant and we didn't know why. Yet starting the workup was a positive step. It gave us both a sense of control and brought us closer together." —An infertility patient, quoted in *The Infertility Book*

Your initial visit to the Texas Center for Reproductive Health starts the evaluation process which is performed by the center's medical director, Samuel P. Marynick, MD, or another physician appropriately trained to perform procedures at the center. The center embryologist, Juan Correa-Pérez, PhD, and the nursing staff may interact with patients during the evaluation.

FEMALE ASSESSMENT

The major part of the assessment is the review of your history and records, particularly the results of your previous tests. This section discusses common tests and diagnostic procedures.

Basal Body Temperature Chart

A basal body temperature chart tracks temperature variations to determine the length of cycles and a probable ovulation date. A woman's temperature usually decreases early in the cycle, dips slightly before ovulation, rises in the luteal phase, and then falls as menstruation begins. The temperature increase coincides with the production of progesterone, the hormone that prepares the uterus for pregnancy. A sample temperature chart is shown in Figure 9.

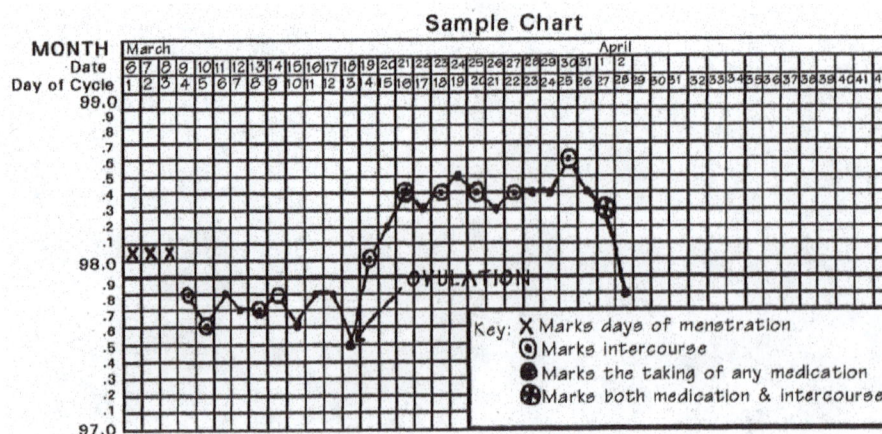

Figure 9. Basal body temperature chart.

Hysterosalpingogram

This x-ray study is used to diagnose tubal blockage or uterine abnormalities and more importantly to tell us the structure of the uterus to allow proper placement of embryos when they are transferred. A physician introduces dye into the uterus through a catheter. As the dye moves through the pelvic organs, an x-ray machine photographs the outlines of the organs as they are revealed by the advancing dye. If the fallopian tubes are open, dye spills out the ends and is later absorbed by the body. If the tubes are blocked, the progress of the dye is halted, and the location of the blockage shows on the x-ray. This test is performed in the first part of the menstrual cycle, the day after all menstrual flow stops. A new form of uterus visualization utilizing ultrasound and saline infusion is called sonohysterography.

Postcoital Test

A postcoital test allows identification of the quality and cellular characteristics of mid-cycle secretions of the cervix and the sperm's reaction to them. Interaction between sperm and cervical mucus plays a critical role in fertility. As ovulation approaches, the mucus should change character and become the consistency of egg white to help sperm swim into the uterus and then into the fallopian tubes. The postcoital test involves a pelvic examination near the time of ovulation, within a few hours following intercourse, to obtain a sample of mucus. The number and movement of sperm are noted, in addition to mucus characteristics.

Serum Progesterone Test and Endometrial Biopsy

These two tests investigate ovarian (corpus luteum) function following egg release and the uterine production of a lining adequate to sustain a fertilized egg. A simple blood test around day 21 of a menstrual cycle measures the level of progesterone. An elevated level suggests adequate ovarian function. An endometrial biopsy is usually done just before menstruation. A patient prepares for the test as if it were a normal pelvic examination. The specialist inserts a small catheter through the cervical canal and retrieves a sample of the uterine lining. After the tissue is fixed and stained in the pathology laboratory, microscopic examination of the tissue should show a mature luteal phase endometrium. Several days are generally required to receive the results of the endometrial biopsy.

Results of the serum progesterone, endometrial biopsy, and postcoital test may reveal problems that exist within the uterus or the ovaries. A fertilized egg may not be able to implant because of a poorly developed endometrial lining. This may be caused by the ovaries not secreting enough progesterone, or the progesterone may not be having the appropriate effect on the uterine lining.

Likewise, cervical mucus or an abnormal cervix may prevent sperm from gaining access to the uterus. A deficiency of sperm in normal cervical mucus suggests the possibility of abnormal semen.

Hormonal Blood Tests

Further investigations may include serum blood tests to check the levels of the hormones that control ovulation:

- ❖ **Estrogen.** A hormone produced by follicles as eggs develop during a menstrual cycle.
- ❖ **Follicle-stimulating hormone (FSH) and luteinizing hormone (LH).** Two hormones that work together to stimulate the ovary and promote growth and development of ovarian follicles that contain eggs.
- ❖ **Prolactin.** A hormone that can adversely affect the influence of FSH on the ovaries if secreted in excess amounts by the pituitary gland.

While compiling complete medical histories, the physician may ask personal questions about lifestyle and sexual habits that have a direct bearing on fertility. (Alcohol, for instance, may retard sperm production in men and decrease fertility in women.) Be honest and straightforward. If you are uncomfortable discussing private subjects, remember we are specialists in the field of fertility treatment. We are experienced in talking to patients about sensitive subjects. And we need you to give accurate and complete information so that we can give you the best treatment.

When your history and records review is complete, the center's physician may give you a physical examination, which may include routine blood tests and a urinalysis.

If appropriate, one or more of the following diagnostic procedures may also be performed as part of the evaluation.

Laparoscopy

This procedure allows a surgeon to view the interior surfaces of the woman's abdomen and reproductive organs. It is used only if other tests have not revealed a reason for ongoing infertility. The procedure is generally uncomplicated and performed as an outpatient surgical procedure. A physician inserts a laparoscope (a long, thin telescope with a light source) through a small incision in the navel to view the reproductive organs. The procedure is performed under general anesthesia.

Sonohysterogram

This is a procedure where under ultrasound monitoring, saline water is injected into the uterus to allow definition of the uterine cavity. Sonohysterography can identify an abnormal uterine cavity.

Hysteroscopy

The hysteroscopy, a cousin to laparoscopy, allows the physician to look inside the uterus. The hysteroscope is a tube-like device with optics which is introduced into the uterus through the cervix without incisions being made and allows visualization of the inside of the uterus. Hysteroscopy is usually performed under general anesthesia in a surgical center as an outpatient procedure. Hysteroscopy may be performed at the center using intravenous sedation on selected patients.

Ultrasound

In this diagnostic procedure, sound waves bounce off internal organs in the abdomen to produce a sonogram, or picture of the uterus and ovaries. A vaginal probe is utilized for ultrasound examinations.

Rubella

If you have not been tested to determine if you are immune to German measles, this test needs to be accomplished before you start an ART cycle.

Autoantibodies

Disorders of the immune system that may cause a woman no demonstrable illness may produce infertility or repeated pregnancy loss. Studies may be requested that assess some of these abnormalities, such as rheumatoid factor, antinuclear antibodies, antithyroid antibodies, antiphospholipid antibodies, or lupus anticoagulant.

Reproductive Immunophenotype and Natural Killer Cell Activation Assay

These studies analyze the makeup and function of the lymphocytes in the woman's blood. Elevation of specific types of white cells is associated with infertility and repeated miscarriage, as is a finding of white cells hyperactivating to antigen stimulus.

Embryotoxicity Assay

This test determines if mouse embryos will grow and develop in the presence of a woman's serum. Serum is blood with the cellular components removed. Embryotoxic substances are associated with infertility and repeated miscarriage.

Additional Tests

It is good if patients involved in ART are shown to have normal levels of iron, vitamin D, zinc, and the hormones related to thyroid function (total T3 and thyroid-stimulating hormone).

MALE ASSESSMENT/ANDROLOGY TESTING

Assessment of the man, like the woman, starts with a review of his history and medical records. After the review, a physical examination and/or further tests as described here may be appropriate.

Physical Examination

The physical examination will include a check of the reproductive organs for abnormalities. The physician will look for a varicocele in the scrotum. This is a common condition that resembles a varicose vein, which can be felt while the patient is standing. A varicocele can affect fertility by decreasing the number of normal sperm produced by the testicles.

Semen Analysis

One of a series of tests now routinely performed at the beginning of fertility treatment is the semen analysis. This test may be performed twice at different points in time because of variability of sperm count and/or sperm production that may be a reflection of illness or stress. After the patient produces a semen sample, laboratory technicians begin testing. Several semen characteristics are evaluated:

❖ **Liquefaction.** Seminal fluid at ejaculation is liquid. Within a few minutes, its consistency changes and it becomes gel-like, then it reliquifies in about 20 to 30 minutes. After it reliquifies, the lab worker measures its volume and begins the analysis.

❖ **Volume.** Too little fluid will result in the sperm having difficulty swimming to the cervical mucus. Too much fluid will dilute the sample, resulting in fewer sperm in a measured volume of liquid.

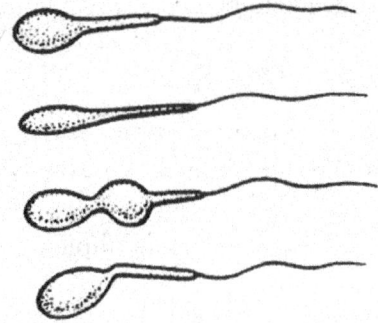

Figure 10. Examples of sperm morphology. From top to bottom: normal sperm, tapered sperm, sperm with mid-piece cytoplasmic inclusion, and sperm with bent mid-piece.

❖ **Viscosity.** This refers to the consistency of the seminal fluid once liquefaction occurs. The sperm swim freely in a flowing liquid but are trapped in thicker fluid. Viscosity is measured on a scale of 0 to 4 with 0 being a normal reading.

❖ **Motility.** Direction and speed determine sperm motility. This analysis identifies what percentage of sperm are normally motile, that is, the fraction that are swimming forward at average to good speed. This should be at least 50% of the total count.

❖ **Morphology.** The shape of the sperm or its morphology is observed because only normal, oval-shaped sperm are able to fertilize an egg (Figure 10).

❖ **Sperm count.** Count is expressed in millions of sperm per cubic centimeter (or milliliter) of volume. A representative volume of the total sperm sample is placed on a grid where the number of sperm can be counted and extrapolated to represent the total population. A count of 40 million is considered good. A low sperm count of fewer than 20 million is known as oligospermia. No sperm count whatsoever is known as azoospermia.

❖ **Agglutination.** If the sperm seem to be sticking together abnormally, they may be reacting to antibodies present in the seminal fluid or to an infection in the male reproductive tract. Sperm that are sticking together will not be available to travel up the female reproductive tract and fertilize eggs.

❖ **Fructose test.** If the semen volume is less than 2 mL, or no sperm are present in the semen, a fructose test is performed. When working properly, the seminal vesicles, small glands that contribute to the semen, add fructose to the semen. Fructose is necessary for normal seminal functioning. Absence of fructose suggests congenital absence of the seminal vesicles or ejaculatory duct obstruction.

Semen Culture

Increased white blood cells in semen may indicate the presence of inflammation and/or infection (e.g., leukocytospermia, bacteriospermia). Performing a semen culture/sensitivity screening may be helpful in determining if certain microorganisms are present in semen. Also, the most efficient and effective medication (e.g., antibiotics) may be determined based on those microbial culture/screening results.

Sperm Antibody Test

Sperm, like a virus or bacteria, can antagonize a man's or woman's immunological system. A small percentage of men and women have antibodies to sperm similar to the immunity developed to a particular disease. The antibodies can show up in vaginal or cervical secretions or in the bloodstream and can kill sperm or cause them to clump together and become incapable of fertilizing an egg. Men can develop antibodies to their own sperm after a vasectomy is performed.

Hormonal Blood Tests

In men, high or low levels of gonadotropin hormones (LH and FSH) may indicate problems with the male reproductive system that need to be investigated.

Microdrop/PXF Testing

This test has been developed at the Texas Center for Reproductive Health and is useful for facilitating sperm identification in cases where azoospermia (no sperm present in the ejaculate) was the original diagnosis. In certain cases (i.e., cryptozoospermia), sperm numbers may be so low that detection via traditional methods is ineffective. In selected cases, the microdrop/PXF technique allows for detection of a sufficient amount of sperm cells to attempt an IVF cycle via the method of intracytoplasmic sperm injection. Furthermore, surgical retrieval of sperm, as with a testicular biopsy, can be avoided in these cases.

Testicular Biopsy

If a semen analysis reveals a very low sperm count or no sperm at all, a biopsy may be performed to determine whether the problem is caused by vas deferens blockage or impaired sperm production. Small pieces of testicular tissue are removed under anesthesia and then examined under a microscope for sperm-generating cells. If the tissue sample shows the absence of sperm-forming cells, infertility may be permanent.

Vasography

This test checks the duct system in the male reproductive tract to locate any obstructions. During this procedure, the patient is put under anesthesia, the scrotum is opened, dye is injected into the duct system, and x-rays are taken to reveal any blockages. Defining an area of obstruction in the vas deferens offers a chance of improving semen if the blockage can be opened with microsurgical techniques.

Rectal Ultrasound

Using a rectal ultrasound probe, a physician experienced in rectal ultrasound can visualize the seminal vesicles and the ejaculatory ducts. If the seminal volume is small, a rectal ultrasound exam may be recommended to assess for ejaculatory duct abnormality.

PROGRAM RECOMMENDATIONS

Based on the results of the evaluation, a center physician will discuss with you whether further testing is needed, if other less sophisticated methods of attempting pregnancy are recommended for you at this point, or if you are ready to enter the Texas Center for Reproductive Health ART program. If you decide to proceed with treatment at the center, the physician will go over which ART therapy is recommended for you.

The Treatment Process

What can you reasonably expect regarding achieving pregnancy through assisted reproductive technology (ART)? There are a number of parts of an ART cycle that must be successfully completed in sequence. The experience of the Texas Center for Reproductive Health and other ART centers has shown the following:

❖ **Egg stimulation** using medications (e.g., Lupron and Gonal-F, Bravelle, or Follistim) to produce multiple follicles is successful in allowing ovum retrieval close to 100% of the time in individuals with normal ovaries. If the ovaries are abnormal or are failing, the success rate drops.

❖ **Following stimulation**, if adequate-sized follicles have developed, the chance of getting the egg from a mature follicle is about 70% to 80%. Generally about seven to nine eggs are collected in the average ART patient.

❖ **Once the eggs are harvested,** they are inseminated. Worldwide, a little more than 50% of the harvested eggs fertilize. Our experience is similar to that of other centers in this regard if there are adequate numbers of normal sperm. If there is a male infertility factor, the rate of fertilization may decrease. When intracytoplasmic sperm injection is used, fertilization occurs on average in most of the normal eggs.

❖ **The chance of pregnancy** occurring with the transfer of normal pre-embryos is related to the age of the woman and the number of pre-embryos transferred. On average, if two to four pre-embryos are transferred, deliveries occur in about 60% of such cases at our center. Generally more embryos are transferred if the patient is older or the embryos are of poor quality. With excellent embryos in a young patient, a single embryo transfer is often performed.

EGG STIMULATION

The process of stimulating egg development begins in the second half of the menstrual cycle prior to the actual ART procedure. You will start monitoring your basal temperature at the beginning of this unassisted cycle. **Notify the nurse when your menses begins**. At this time an appointment will be made for you and your partner. If you do not have spontaneous periods (or if you have an artificial cycle stimulation), you will be given a 4-week cycle of Premarin and Provera or an oral contraceptive pill to regulate your menstrual cycle. In such a cycle, Lupron would be started on day 21 of the Premarin/Provera or oral contraceptive regimen.

In a natural cycle, your temperature chart will be evaluated following ovulation, your progesterone blood level will be determined, and an ultrasound will be performed.

If adequate progesterone is present in your bloodstream (which signifies previous ovulation), Lupron will be started daily at a dose of 0.5 to 1 mg (0.1–0.2 mL) per day. Lupron is given as a subcutaneous injection. Lupron is a compound that suppresses your pituitary gland from producing follicle-stimulating hormone (FSH) and luteinizing hormone (LH), which stimulate the ovaries to develop eggs. Timing is critical here. Lupron is effective in suppressing pituitary function only after ovulation has occurred. If Lupron is given and ovulation has not occurred, Lupron can stimulate the pituitary gland to release LH and FSH. Such a response would be exactly the opposite of what is desired. Lupron helps to prevent a "premature" LH surge before the follicles are adequately mature, which would end the entire ART cycle. Cancellation of a cycle due to a premature LH surge previously occurred in about 10% of the cases. With Lupron, that cancellation rate has been reduced to less than 5%. You can expect a menstrual period to begin 7 to 10 days following the start of Lupron. A nurse will help you and your partner learn how to administer the injections you will need during this phase of the treatment program. She will also go over the program calendar so that you are prepared for each required activity.

Prior to leaving the center, a return visit for you and your partner will be scheduled to begin FSH or human menopausal gonadotropin (hMG) therapy. Your partner will be requested to collect one or more semen samples for cryopreservation (freezing). By cryopreserving a semen sample, we ensure that if a sample of adequate quality is not obtained on the day of egg retrieval, we will still be able to attempt fertilization of collected eggs using the frozen semen sample.

Other blood tests that will be required of you and your partner are HIV (AIDS) and hepatitis. This is for your protection and the protection of your potential offspring and our staff. The male will be instructed on how to provide a semen sample. The quality of the sample is best if ejaculation occurred 48 hours before the sample to be analyzed is collected.

Your next appointment at the center will take place approximately 10 days after starting Lupron. At this appointment, an ultrasound examination of the ovaries will be performed, an estradiol level measured, and the depth of your uterus measured with a small catheter (only if this measurement has not been previously performed). This procedure is called a trial transfer, and this measurement is important for accurately placing pre-embryos on the day of pre-embryo transfer.

FSH or hMG therapy will be started at this point. hMG, a medication made up of FSH and LH, and FSH alone stimulate the ovaries to produce follicles. There are several brand names for FSH and hMG. Administration of these medications will be taught to you and your husband. All medications are given intramuscularly or subcutaneously. Most women begin on a set protocol of medication for 3 days (see IVF calendar). The injections will be given each evening at a time that is convenient for you. If more than three ampules of medication are given, the medication will be divided into morning and evening dosages.

From day 4 of medication, the dose will be adjusted according to your follicular development and estradiol values. Appointments to the center will generally occur at 2- to 3-day intervals during morning hours. This allows your physician to have the day's testing back before deciding if the dose of medication needs to be adjusted.

Stimulation medication is continued daily, as is Lupron, until an adequate number of follicles more than 18 mm in diameter develop. Generally, at least six mature follicles are present at this stage, though there is variation in this number. When stimulation medication is given, one problem that can occur is hyperstimulation of the ovaries. In hyperstimulation, the ovaries become enlarged and produce some discomfort. Generally, hyperstimulation is not serious in patients undergoing in vitro fertilization with embryo transfer (IVF/ET). However, severe hyperstimulation (which is not common) may necessitate hospitalization and possibly treatment to remove fluid that has built up in the abdomen and rarely is fatal.

When enough follicles mature, an injection of human chorionic gonadotropin (hCG) is given to complete the maturation process. The hCG dosage is usually 10,000 units, to be administered in the late evening. You will be given a specific time to administer this injection. **Please give the injection at the appointed time.** If you do not, please let the nurse coordinator know as soon as possible. **It is critical to retrieve the follicles 34 to 35 hours after the hCG injection.** If you miss your assigned time, the nurse coordinator must try to reschedule your retrieval to accommodate that timing requirement.

When scheduling the egg retrieval procedure, the nurse coordinator goes over in detail what will happen and what you need to do. Women are advised not to eat or drink anything after midnight before the procedure. The couple should plan on arriving at the center 45 minutes before the procedure is scheduled to begin. This time is required for the woman to change into a surgical gown and be sedated.

This is an exciting time. If you feel strung like a piano wire, do not be surprised. Couples can deal with the ups and downs of treatment through mutual love and support, as well as a reasonable set of expectations. Remember, it was not long ago that this procedure was not even an option. You are among a generation of couples who now can hope for their own child.

Getting to egg retrieval can be a memorable trip. As one mother of an in vitro baby said:

> *One of the most difficult things I went through was the roller coaster ride waiting for estradiol levels. Would it be high enough? Would I have enough eggs? Would I be on another day of stimulation? It was really the most exhausting part of the process.* —An infertility patient, quoted in *From Infertility to In Vitro Fertilization*

In the unlikely event your IVF/ET cycle needs to be discontinued, don't be too discouraged. It does not mean that future cycles will end with the same results. We often learn valuable information in a canceled cycle that improves the result of a subsequent cycle.

Injection sites need a rest between shots. Your nurse coordinator can help you establish a site rotation plan. Rotating the placement of shots will help you minimize discomfort. A warm bath can do wonders for sore injection sites and jangled nerves. If an injection site is irritated, warm compresses may ease the discomfort.

If an injection site becomes painful and develops a hard knot-like texture, this needs to be brought to the attention of a nurse or a physician.

Texas Center for Reproductive Health
(214) 821-2274
Please use the following log for permanent record of your IVF/ET cycle

IVF/ET LOG		
	DATES	**NOTES**
1. Menstrual period begins—notify center and begin recording daily basal temperature. Please do not engage in unprotected sexual intercourse.		
2. Blood tests—HIV, hepatitis, rubella, and any other special-ordered tests.		
3. Semen analysis and backup frozen semen sample—2 days abstinence prior to collection.		
4. Antibiotic taken by couple for 10 days, to begin day 3 of menses.		
5. Schedule hysterosalpingogram to be done day 7 to 10 of menses.		
6. Sonogram prior to initiation of Lupron, luteal day 7.		
7. Begin daily Lupron 0.2 mL (or as specified for your particular case) **subcutaneously** in p.m. if progesterone level is adequate.		
8. Menstrual flow usually day 7 to 10 on Lupron.		
9. Trial transfer, sonogram and estradiol prior to beginning stimulation. Do not exercise vigorously after beginning stimulation therapy.		

LUPRON*	hMG	FSH	DATE	ESTRADIOL
0.2 ml	amps	amps		
0.1 ml	amps	amps		
0.1 ml	amps	amps		
0.1 ml	amps	amps		
0.1 ml	amps	amps		
0.1 ml	amps	amps		
0.1 ml	amps	amps		
0.1 ml	amps	amps		
0.1 ml	amps	amps		
0.1 ml	amps	amps		
0.1 ml	amps	amps		

* Dose may vary depending on your specific case.

Reconstitution of hMG or FSH

1 glass ampule hMG or
FSH powder equals
one dose

1 glass ampule sterile
saline (salt water)
equals 2 cc (mL) liquid

hMG and FSH may come 10 ampules to a box with 10 glass ampules of sterile normal saline (salt water). Some hMG and FSH brands are packaged as single ampules for injection, while some brands are packaged as multidose vials or multidose syringes.

Formula to Reconstitute hMG or FSH

1 amp hMG or FSH mixed with ½ cc sterile saline.

2 amps hMG or FSH mixed with ½ cc sterile saline.

3 amps hMG or FSH mixed with ½ cc sterile saline.

4 or 5 amps hMG or FSH mixed with 1 cc sterile saline.

If greater than 3 amps of medication are needed in one day, individual instructions will be given, and part of the daily medication will be in the morning and part in the evening.

IVF/ET TABLE			
	TIME	DATE	NOTES
STOP LUPRON, hMG, AND/OR FSH; take hCG injection; urinalysis and hematocrit required; review written preoperative directions			
Egg retrieval; semen collection; review written postoperative and pretransfer directions			
Embryo transfer; review written post-transfer directions			
Bedrest; continue progesterone IM as directed. For some patients, progesterone dose is 100 mg daily. Progesterone may vary for specific patients.		to	
		to	
Pregnancy test			
Post conference			
Sonogram to confirm pregnancy			

EGG RETRIEVAL—IVF/ET

IVF/ET involves removing eggs from the female's ovaries and placing them in a sterile liquid (a medium) with the male's sperm to let the natural process of fertilization take place outside the womb, in vitro (in glass).

Our center medical team will perform your egg retrieval. In the IVF/ET process, egg retrieval is generally done in the early morning. **Remember not to eat or drink anything after midnight before the procedure**. Arrive at the center 45 minutes before the retrieval is scheduled.

When you arrive, you and your partner will be given head and shoe covers. Your partner will remain in the recovery room. Your doctor will be in to talk with you and your partner before the retrieval to answer any questions you may have. You will walk into the retrieval suite, where EKG pads will be placed on your chest, a pulse oximeter will be placed on one of your fingers to check your heartbeat, and a blood pressure cuff will be secured to an arm. An IV will be used to give you medications during the surgery to prevent pain and anxiety.

Your legs are placed in supports on the operating table, in a position similar to that for a pelvic exam. Your vagina is cleansed with embryo culture medium. Once the vagina is cleansed, a Foley catheter is placed to drain your bladder of urine. Then the ultrasound probe is inserted into the vagina. Using the ultrasound scan as a guide, the physician passes a needle through the top of the vagina and into the ovary. The physician locates the follicles in each ovary and harvests an egg from each follicle.

Harvesting is accomplished by puncturing the follicle, then suctioning (or aspirating) the fluid out through the needle into a sterile container. The follicle is flushed with egg-collecting medium liquid. The containers of follicular fluid are handed to the embryologist, who evaluates the fluid for the presence of eggs. On average, an egg is collected from every two of three mature follicles harvested.

Once all the follicles have been aspirated, the ultrasound probe is removed, and you are taken to a couple's recovery room. There, you rejoin your partner and will stay lying still until the analgesia has worn off to the point where you are awake and able to return home. This usually takes about 2 to 3 hours. The physician will be able to tell you the number of eggs retrieved and their quality (Figure 11). You should not sign important documents or drive a car or operate dangerous equipment for the remainder of the day of egg retrieval. Prior to leaving the center, you may receive an injection of progesterone in oil to begin the preparation of the uterine lining for embryo transfer. Getting past egg retrieval can give couples a real feeling of accomplishment.

"There's something comforting about hearing how many eggs you've produced."
—An IVF patient

Good egg—
clear uniform cytoplasm

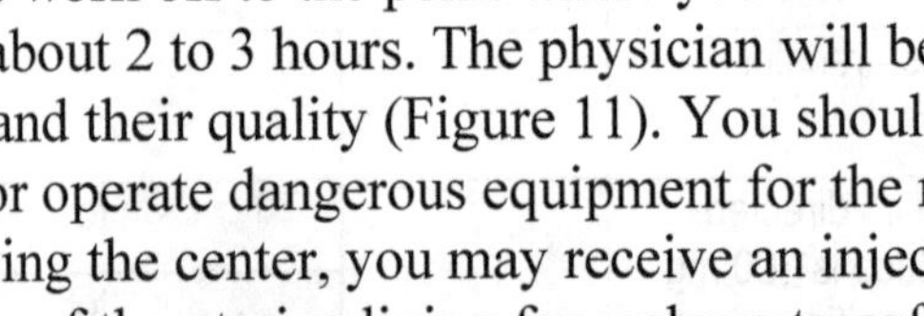

Egg of questionable quality—
irregular darkened cytoplasm

Figure 11. Comparison of egg quality.

SEMEN PREPARATION

To maximize the opportunities for fertilization, it will be necessary for the husband to produce a semen sample which is processed before being utilized to fertilize eggs. The semen sample will be collected after the time of egg retrieval. The quality of the sample is best if there was an ejaculation 48 hours before the sample is collected.

Masturbation is the acceptable method of collection. Because sexually arousing material improves the quality of a semen sample collected by masturbation, such material is provided in the semen collection room.

Before you collect the sample, be sure to wash your hands with soap and water and wash your penis using only water **(no soap)** thoroughly with the foreskin pulled back if you are not circumcised. If you are not circumcised, leave the foreskin back until the sample is obtained.

The sample is collected into a sterile container. When the sample has been collected, put the top securely back on the collection container, being careful not to touch the inside of the container or the lid. Refer to specific instructions that will be provided in the collection room.

As soon as the sample is collected, please notify the center laboratory using the call bell in the collection room. When brought to the laboratory, the sample is processed in preparation for fertilization. First, the semen is placed across a separation gradient or other suitable processing method. The separation gradient is a molecular filter which allows sperm to migrate through the molecular filter when force is applied to the sample using a centrifuge. Bacteria, white blood cells, dead sperm, and other particulate matter in the semen do not migrate well through a molecular filter and are thereby separated from the motile sperm. Next capacitation medium is added to the sperm. The capacitation medium maximizes the sperm's ability to penetrate the wife's eggs.

After separation, the quantity of sperm is calculated. For IVF treatment, about 50,000 motile sperm are added per egg. If the sperm quality is poor but there is an abundant quantity, up to 500,000 sperm will be added per egg to increase the likelihood of egg fertilization, or the intracytoplasmic sperm injection (ICSI) technique may be used instead. The preferred insemination method at the Texas Center for Reproductive Health is ICSI, due to the higher fertilization rates obtained.

A sample of semen is frozen or cryopreserved prior to starting an ART cycle. This frozen sample may be used for egg fertilization if the husband is unavailable or ill the day of egg retrieval or if the semen sample collected the day of egg retrieval is considered inadequate for a reasonable chance of egg fertilization.

STANDARD IN VITRO FERTILIZATION

After eggs are retrieved from ovarian follicles, each is viewed under a microscope and graded. Mature eggs receive a top grade. Immature eggs receive a lower score and are incubated for 24 hours to improve their chance of fertilization. However, immature eggs may not continue to develop. A degenerated egg is dead and will not fertilize.

Eggs are cultured in plastic containers, using a special fluid free of bacteria called an insemination medium. This medium provides an environment in which eggs and pre-embryos can mature and develop. Eggs remain inside an incubator prior to, during, and after fertilization.

About 5 to 6 hours after egg retrieval, sperm are added to each egg-holding container. The male's sperm sample has been processed in the laboratory prior to fertilization. Now surrounded by 50,000 to 500,000 swimming sperm, each egg is returned to the incubator. In unassisted reproduction, an egg would be exposed to about 500 sperm. Fertilization actually starts occurring within the first few hours after natural ovulation or after sperm are placed with an egg in vitro.

Sometimes with IVF, as in nature, when eggs and sperm meet, fertilization does not occur. With good sperm, approximately 60% to 70% of inseminated eggs will fertilize. However, if most or all of the eggs fail to fertilize, another fertility problem may exist. This allows IVF to be used as a diagnostic tool to identify an egg fertilization problem that would otherwise not have been discovered.

For those eggs that are fertilized, the next step is the process of cell division called cleavage. This will begin several hours after fertilization.

Once cleavage has begun, the zygote may continue to divide at regular intervals. Usually, cell division indicates a healthy pre-embryo that has a possibility to implant. When the fastest growing pre-embryos reach four to eight cells, they may be transferred (Figure 12). On occasion an egg may fertilize but fail to divide, or it may divide several times and then cellular division stops. In either of these cases, the fertilized egg cannot produce a pregnancy.

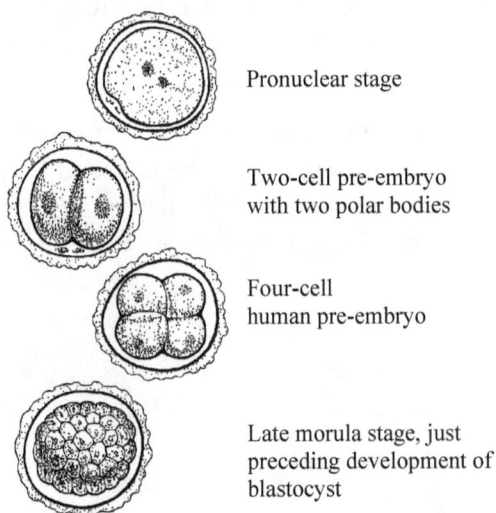

Pronuclear stage

Two-cell pre-embryo
with two polar bodies

Four-cell
human pre-embryo

Late morula stage, just
preceding development of
blastocyst

Figure 12. Growth stages of human pre-embryo.

Presently, we prefer to monitor the pre-embryos in the laboratory for 3 to 5 days to allow for transfer of the one to three embryos most likely to implant.

INTRACYTOPLASMIC SPERM INJECTION

If there are few normal sperm, if the sperm have reduced motility, if failure to conceive is unexplained, or if there has been an abnormally low rate of fertilization in a previous cycle, intracytoplasmic sperm injection (ICSI) may be used to seek to enhance egg fertilization.

In ICSI, a solitary sperm is injected into an egg using a microscopic glass needle. Fertilization rates with ICSI generally exceed 75%, if the eggs are normal. ICSI is the preferred insemination method at Texas Center for Reproductive Health.

NUMBER OF EMBRYOS TRANSFERRED

Prior to embryo transfer, couples must decide how many embryos they wish to return to the uterus. The Texas Center for Reproductive Health will transfer a maximum of two pre-embryos for most couples. This maximum was established to provide the best chance of conception while minimizing the possibility of high-risk multiple pregnancy. The incidence of twins through IVF is about one out of every four pregnancies; triplets, less than one out of 20 cases; and quadruplets, approximately one out of every 1000 cases. A maximum of five pre-embryos may be transferred to couples when the woman is 39 years or older and in most cases where three previous IVF/ET cycles have not resulted in a pregnancy. In younger couples, transfers may be limited to one or two pre-embryos.

If more pre-embryos develop than can be transferred, the Texas Center for Reproductive Health offers couples the opportunity to freeze and store extra pre-embryos to be thawed and transferred in an unstimulated cycle at a later time. Embryo freezing is discussed in more detail in the Cryopreservation section (p. 35). Please review this information on cryopreservation thoroughly, because your decision on whether or not to use this option must be made prior to the transfer procedure.

On the day following egg retrieval, a member of the nursing staff, an embryologist, or your physician will call you to report the progress of your pre-embryos and to schedule embryo transfer, usually within 72 to 120 hours of egg retrieval.

Waiting for that call from the staff to hear about the success of the embryo development can produce some anxiety. Rest assured you will be called with this information, and you should try to remain calm. Although it is important now to spend time together, both of you should reserve some moments alone for peace and reflection.

MICROMANIPULATION

For those couples who would be unlikely to achieve pregnancy through conventional IVF/ET, we offer procedures referred to as gamete micromanipulation. In gamete micromanipulation, the sperm and/or egg are manipulated using very small glass pipettes and/or glass needles. The purpose of these procedures may be to selectively place a sperm into the egg cytoplasm, i.e., intracytoplasmic sperm injection or ICSI.

For couples who have had previous IVF/ET where normal embryos were placed in the uterus but a pregnancy did not result, we may recommend a subsequent IVF/ET cycle with assisted embryo hatching. In this procedure the egg is allowed to fertilize. Following fertilization, the pre-embryo is micromanipulated to produce an opening in the zona pellucida or eggshell. Producing this opening in the eggshell aids the "hatching" of the pre-embryo and its implantation into the uterus to establish a pregnancy.

In these procedures (ICSI and assisted pre-embryo hatching), the egg or pre-embryo is held by a small glass pipette called a holding pipette. The sperm is directly injected into the egg using manipulation with a glass needle (ICSI) and the embryo shell is opened using a glass knife to divide the eggshell.

Micromanipulation procedures are very technical and difficult to perform and require much practice to learn. These procedures are potentially helpful in certain cases, but agreement to have these procedures performed on your gametes brings potential risks. Micromanipulation of an egg or pre-embryo may be fatal to that egg or embryo. Thus, these procedures may result in loss of eggs or pre-embryos that have been produced.

Other problems that occur relate to the chance that ICSI will not produce fertilization of the egg. Even if a sperm is successfully injected into an egg, the sperm and egg must still undergo the complex process of fertilization, which requires normal functioning eggs, and this may occur in less than 50% of ICSI eggs in some cases because the egg, the sperm, or both do not function normally.

Fertilization may result in the egg carrying more than one set of chromosomes (polyploidy). A pre-embryo that contains excess chromosome material will not be viable. If ICSI results in a normal pre-embryo and if normal pre-embryos are placed into the uterus, delivery rates currently are 50% to 60% per cycle.

Likewise, assisted hatching may be lethal to a pre-embryo. If assisted hatching is successfully accomplished and a normal pre-embryo with an opened zona pellucida is placed in the uterus, pregnancy rates currently are more than 50% per cycle in women less than 40 years old.

GENETIC SCREENING OF EMBRYOS

Genetic screening of embryos—preimplantation genetic diagnosis and preimplantation genetic screening—are techniques that are gaining worldwide acceptance. The most common applications involve (1) single gene testing (e.g., cystic fibrosis), (2) aneuploidy screening, and (3) sex chromosome screening (i.e., family balancing). By using these techniques, we can select healthy embryos for transfer and/or cryopreservation and avoid choosing those embryos that may be genetically abnormal.

Genetic testing involves micromanipulation of the embryo(s) to obtain cells on day 3 of development. Embryos must reach a cleavage stage of at least 6 cells before being suitable for biopsy. The biopsied cells are sent to a genetics lab for testing, and the results are generally available 36 hours later. The genetic report is reviewed by the embryologist, and embryo(s) are chosen for transfer based on those results and the quality of the embryo(s).

EMBRYO TRANSFER

Embryo transfer will normally occur 72 to 120 hours after ovum retrieval when the pre-embryos are at approximately the eight cell to blastocyst stage of development.

At the center, the woman will take a small amount of tranquilizer to become more relaxed for the procedure. Arrive at the center about 45 minutes before the transfer. We strongly encourage you to experience this procedure as a couple. Both of you will be brought into the transfer suite wearing head and shoe covers. The woman should not drive a motor vehicle or sign important documents for 24 hours after she has taken the pre-transfer tranquilizer.

While you prepare for embryo transfer, your pre-embryos are placed in the mobile IVF cart in culture medium. Both partners will be shown pictures of the pre-embryos (taken through the microscope) prior to the transfer. The pre-embryos are then placed in a thin, flexible transfer catheter.

The transfer process is similar to a regular pelvic examination, and no anesthesia is necessary. A speculum will be inserted into the vagina and the cervix will be cleansed. It may be necessary to place a suture in the cervix to stabilize it. The physician performing the embryo transfer will then aspirate or use swabs to remove mucus from the cervix. Next, the physician will thread the catheter through the cervix into the uterus. Pre-embryos will be gently placed at the top of the uterus. On occasion, more than one attempt at transfer is required if the transfer catheter cannot be positioned within 1 to 3 minutes. It has been found that pregnancy rates do not differ whether embryo transfer occurs on the first or subsequent attempts. In cases where the cervix is narrowed, it may be necessary to dilate the cervix prior to transfer. Cervical dilation doesn't influence pregnancy rate. The embryo transfer may be visualized using ultrasound monitoring, in which case the wife will need a full bladder at the time of transfer.

Following embryo transfer, the transfer catheter is checked to make sure no embryo(s) are retained in the catheter. If one or more embryos are retained in the catheter, the remaining embryos are transferred to the place in the uterus utilized for the initial transfer. On completion of the transfer, center personnel will move you from the pelvic exam position to lying on the transfer bed. During this repositioning, it is important for you to relax your muscles and to relax in general.

With day 3 transfer, pre-embryos enter the uterus at an earlier stage than they do naturally. Normally, pre-embryos spend several days moving through the fallopian tubes before reaching the uterus.

After the transfer you remain on a bed in the transfer suite, which is quiet with dimmed lights. You need to rest and remain on your back for approximately 1 hour. If you have a full bladder at transfer, you will be allowed to empty your bladder about 15 to 30 minutes following embryo transfer. Tension can cause the body to release hormones that contract the uterus, and this may decrease the chance of embryo implantation. Husbands are encouraged to be with their wives throughout the rest period. A lounge chair is provided in the transfer suite for his use. Your first pregnancy test is scheduled 14 days following egg retrieval. You will be released and taken to your car in a wheelchair after the post-transfer rest period. Remember, you should not drive a motor vehicle or operate dangerous equipment or sign important documents for 24 hours following embryo transfer.

AFTER THE TRANSFER

You will be on complete bed rest except for meals and bathroom breaks for 3 days after the transfer. You will continue resting with limited activity within the home for the next 7 days. You must not do anything strenuous the 2 weeks following the transfer. If the pregnancy tests are positive, you will need to continue to avoid strenuous activity.

In the time between the retrieval and the first pregnancy test, you will generally be taking daily progesterone injections. Progesterone supports the lining of the uterus and helps mature the lining to enhance its ability to allow an embryo to implant and maintain a pregnancy, so it is extremely important that you take these injections as they are recommended. Also, you may take one injection of hCG during this time as instructed on the ART calendar. **You should not have intercourse between the time of your 10,000 IU of hCG and the first pregnancy test.** If the first pregnancy test is positive, further abstinence from intercourse may be recommended to let the embryo "get a good start."

During the 7 to 12 days between embryo transfer and the first beta hCG pregnancy test, you will be on an emotional roller coaster ride. Do not, however, do any physical exercise; instead, do mental activities that interest you. Pamper yourself. You may want to watch videos, read books, work crossword puzzles, do needlepoint, or write letters.

On day 14 post-retrieval, a pregnancy test is performed. This sensitive blood test can detect a pregnancy at the earliest possible time. The laboratory checks for the presence of hCG, a substance produced by a developing placenta, which is detectable in the bloodstream. If the hCG test is positive, a follow-up test to confirm the results of the first test will be done 2 days later. A third test will be done about a week after the first test. A continuing rise in hCG confirms a progressing pregnancy. A prenatal vitamin with folic acid will also be prescribed during the ART cycle and continued if the hCG test is positive.

If pregnancy is confirmed to be progressing, after the third hCG, you will schedule an appointment to return in 3 weeks for an ultrasound exam to confirm a gestational sac. During this time you will continue taking daily progesterone injections. At 6 weeks post–egg retrieval, if the ultrasound exam confirms a viable fetus in a gestational sac within the uterus, you may be switched to vaginal progesterone or oral progesterone daily until about week 12 to 18 of the pregnancy. Normal prenatal care with your obstetrician should begin after an ultrasound at 8 weeks. Your doctor at the center generally continues as a consultant with your obstetrician regarding the pregnancy and the reduction of supplemental progesterone. Do not discontinue supplemental progesterone unless this is approved by the center physician.

If your ART procedure fails, you should take some time to cope with your disappointment. Failure to conceive is not a reflection on you as a person or your ability to be a parent. You may wish to try again. For many couples, a second or third IVF cycle has as likely a chance of success as the first. The father of a 1-month-old son born through IVF said:

"I would encourage everyone definitely to maintain a positive attitude. The hardest part of the whole procedure is dealing with failure. And it's inevitable that you're going to have a few failures, and after a while you just stop wanting to try because you don't want to fail again. If you could just keep it in perspective and know that in vitro fertilization is a trial-and-error scientific procedure and sometimes you just have to expect problems, that will help a great deal."
—Quoted in *From Infertility to In Vitro Fertilization*

CRYOPRESERVATION

Prior to IVF/ET, we will request that the male collect one (or more) semen samples for cryopreservation. By cryopreserving a semen sample, we ensure that if a sample of adequate quality is not obtained on the day of egg retrieval, we will still be able to attempt fertilization of collected eggs.

Embryo cryopreservation is simply pre-embryo freezing. Pregnancy rates in IVF are directly related to the number of embryos transferred. However, multiple pregnancies increase dramatically when more than two pre-embryos are returned to the woman. To minimize the risk of producing a multiple order pregnancy, if more than two pre-embryos develop, extra pre-embryos can be frozen and preserved to be placed in a future cycle.

Cryopreservation has several advantages:

❖ During an ART cycle, excess eggs can be cryopreserved if a couple does not wish to produce a large number of embryos or eggs can be inseminated and extra embryos placed in cryostorage.
❖ Additional egg retrieval in a later assisted cycle is thereby unnecessary. Pre-embryos that were developed in an earlier cycle can be cryopreserved and then transferred during a second cycle at a later point in time.
❖ Embryos can be transferred during a cycle free of fertility medication (a natural cycle).
❖ Embryos can be transferred during a hormone-supported cycle. In these cycles hormones are given to mimic a normal cycle.

The primary risk associated with cryopreservation is that the pre-embryo may not be able to survive freeze-thaw, which occurs about 10% of the time. At this time, the likelihood of pregnancy from cryopreserved pre-embryos transferred to the uterus at our center is about 50% to 60% when one or two pre-embryos (that look normal after thawing) are placed into the uterus.

Cryopreservation Issues

Examine your personal convictions about suspending the development of a pre-embryo through cryopreservation. Your own moral compass must guide you. Cryopreservation may not be ethically acceptable to you, which means you must consider whether to fertilize only a portion of the eggs retrieved or to fertilize all available eggs. Most religious denominations have not yet formed a policy regarding this new technological development. If you feel any uncertainty, we suggest that you consult with your clergyman for guidance.

Because cryopreservation is relatively new in the United States, law is still being written on the status of frozen pre-embryos. Perhaps the most famous case dealing with this issue involved a couple in Australia who died in a car crash, leaving embryos in frozen storage at an infertility clinic. Who inherited the dead couple's estate? Did the embryos constitute heirs? If they did, who were their guardians? The questions were endless and difficult to answer.

Texas Center for Reproductive Health has developed its own policies, philosophies, and consent forms to avoid confusion in the area of sperm, eggs, and pre-embryo cryopreservation. Please read the consent forms carefully and ask any questions you might have. Texas Center for Reproductive Health only works with committed couples in an ART procedure. In the case of divorce, death, or mental incapacity of a partner, the Texas Center for Reproductive Health will abide by your consent documents and applicable law to determine the final disposition of the pre-embryos.

Treatment Review

No matter what the outcome, couples will meet with a center physician to review treatment. It may be helpful for you to go over notations in this workbook before attending this meeting. That way you can be sure to get answers to all of your questions.

The physician may discuss:

- ❖ Your initial diagnosis
- ❖ Response to stimulation
- ❖ Follicle development prior to/at egg retrieval
- ❖ Ovum fertilization
- ❖ Embryo transfer
- ❖ Recommendations

Please help us evaluate the Texas Center for Reproductive Health. Think about these questions prior to the treatment review and bring up any issues of importance to you—whether negative or positive.

1. Did you have any trouble administering injections? Did you receive enough instruction?

2. Did staff report each test result in a timely manner? Were results explained to you in terms you could understand?

3. Were you comfortable with ultrasound-guided egg retrieval? Was it what you expected?

4. Did relaxation techniques suggested in the *Couple's Workbook* help you to better cope with the treatment process?

5. Were you comfortable in your treatment?

6. Did you find the *Couple's Workbook* useful in preparing for treatment? How would you change it?

7. Were you comfortable with our staff? Did they offer support and understanding?

If you have any comments you would like to make regarding your treatment, please let us know. We want our patients to have the best experience possible at the Texas Center for Reproductive Health. Your feedback will help us achieve that goal.

Coping with Stress

An infertile woman sat in a reproductive medicine specialist's office distressed with her inability to have a child, crying until her eyes were swollen and her tissue supply exhausted. The doctor listened quietly, watching as she filled one tissue after another with tears. Suddenly, the woman turned cold eyes on the doctor, telling him he was the last in a long line of specialists she was going to subject herself to. Just what did he have to offer that the others didn't and could he guarantee she would become pregnant? Anger swept the doctor's face and he pushed the tissue box over to the woman. He said, "Cry some more until you can't cry any more. Then let's go down the corridor to a room where a woman who has 6 weeks to live is dying. Then maybe we can keep all this in perspective."

When the woman related this story, she did so without any malice toward the doctor. She admitted he told her not what she wanted to hear but what she needed to hear. Infertility treatment had taken over her life. She could not see over it, under it, or around it. He helped her lift her head up so she could see the whole landscape, not just the potholes in the road.

Each of us will experience crises in our lives that we feel we cannot endure. For you, infertility may be your first major life obstacle. Those who come through crises intact use resources within themselves, their communities, their families, and friends.

Learn More

Be an active partner in your treatment. Follow your workup closely and ask questions if you do not understand where your doctor is headed with your treatment. Read about reproduction, infertility, and fertility. Know your own case thoroughly. Learn the jargon you hear in the office. Search the Internet and visit the library. The more you know, the less likely you are to overlook important options, according to Dr. Baruch Fischhoff, who studies the decision-making process at Carnegie Mellon University in Pittsburgh. However, be careful about accepting as truth all you read or hear. **The Internet is not policed, and neither are books or newspapers**. Also, there are individuals who have little or no training in this area who are full of information that has no foundation in truth.

Remember You Are Not Alone

Talking about a problem makes it easier to tackle. Being part of a support group can help shrink infertility down to size. Along with the tears you shed, there's a lot of laughter, too. Resolve, a national organization for infertile couples, has chapters throughout the United States, including Dallas/Fort Worth. A membership gives you invaluable information about medical care, contact with other infertile couples, and general references on your condition. You will find much comfort in knowing there are others like yourself who are suffering with a fertility problem.

Visit your minister or clergyman or talk to family members about your feelings. You may be surprised how many people within your family have experienced the same disappointment. Infertility does not come up in casual conversation; the subject must be deliberately broached.

A professional counselor who specializes in treating infertile couples says she tries to help couples appreciate what they already have—a strong marriage that welcomes children. One couple takes time out each Valentine's Day to remember why they want children so desperately—because of the love they feel for each other.

Don't Be Afraid To Ask for Help

It shows strength, not weakness, to admit a problem is too big to handle alone. Texas Center for Reproductive Health can refer you to counselors who are experienced in dealing with anxiety related to infertility. Do not hesitate to ask. If you would like to talk with other patients who are undergoing the same kind of therapy, contact Resolve for names of members who will be pleased to help you.

Keep a Journal ·

One patient who underwent in vitro fertilization, became pregnant, and then miscarried credits her journal with saving her sanity. Although tears accompanied every word she wrote, she poured her feelings onto paper. Writing and crying, writing and crying, she helped to heal herself.

Often jotting down your feelings relieves tension and reduces the problem in size and complexity. Feelings of depression can be eased. If for no other reason than to try it, begin a journal at the outset of your ART cycle.

Sometimes You Gain More by Giving

Begin with your spouse. Infertility is a time of persistent stress. Besides normal daily problems, couples must decide about tests, treatment, medication, surgery, or advanced technologies. Communication may become increasingly difficult.

Guilt and anger are common feelings. Disagreements will happen; tempers will flare. Try to listen to each other. Support and respect one another. Take care of your relationship. Your quality of life is important now. By being honest, caring, and respectful of each other, you can find answers. That means fighting fair along the road to resolution. Reason together fairly and compassionately.

One coping method suggested by Barbara Eck Menning, founder of Resolve, is the **20-minute rule.** The woman is usually the more verbal and emotional partner, no matter who has the problem. To help keep infertility from being the sole subject of discussion in a household, set aside a period each evening to talk about infertility. Using a timer, limit each person to 20 minutes. First one person speaks, then the other. The person not speaking is expected to listen. This technique is particularly helpful in achieving these outcomes:

- ❖ The woman will talk less about infertility and will be more succinct.
- ❖ The man is more willing to listen because he is assured of an end point.
- ❖ The woman feels she has an interested listener and is supported. Both may feel relieved to see the other feeling better.
- ❖ The rest of the evening may be spent in other, more pleasant, pursuits.
- ❖ As the woman talks less, the man may feel inclined to talk more. Sometimes, according to Eck Menning, the woman has been grieving for two.

Humor Helps

It is important for you as a couple and as individuals to exercise your sense of humor. Laughter may not always be the best medicine, but it is consistently an effective one, a tremendous tension-reliever.

- ❖ When looking for a movie, pick a comedy or a light adventure.
- ❖ Try going to a comedy club to see live entertainers, or watch a comedy show on television. (There's plenty to choose from!)
- ❖ Spend time with friends or relatives whose company you particularly enjoy.

One infertile man tells the story of a comic discussion that began in his infertility support group about what sort of container makes an ideal vessel for transporting semen. Everyone in the room agreed that a mayonnaise jar made a teaspoonful of semen look too pathetic. On the other hand, they thought perfume bottles were impossible to hit and too effeminate. Used caviar jars or artichoke heart jars were just the right size, but they seemed too pretentious. What the group decided was the perfect jar to deliver a semen specimen was an item that no infertile couple would have around the house: an empty baby food jar.

Financial Considerations

"When you really want children, you set your priorities. We think babies are more important than fancy vacations or a boat. We were able to budget for in vitro fertilization. But we're sorry that insurance doesn't usually cover it because a lot of couples just can't spend the money to go through these procedures."
—An infertility patient, quoted in *From Infertility to In Vitro Fertilization*

Investing in a family can reap priceless rewards. But the costs of advanced technologies, such as in vitro fertilization, are still borne primarily by couples. Insurance companies may specifically exclude this procedure from coverage.

In Texas, a bill passed in 1987 requiring insurance companies, health maintenance organizations, and preferred provider organizations to offer the option of coverage for in vitro fertilization to customers, group or individual, at each annual renewal period. The offer must be rejected in writing.

Owners of small businesses who have direct control over the purchase of group health insurance and individual subscribers benefit most from this change in the Texas Insurance Code. Although insurance carriers must make an offer to large companies with group health plans, the offer can be rejected without consultation with employees. Self-insured companies are exempt from the mandate because they are regulated by federal statute.

GENERAL ATTITUDE TOWARD COVERAGE OF ART PROCEDURES

Private Health Insurance

According to a recent managed care survey, only 13% of insurance companies pay for IVF. Companies that do not pay for in vitro fertilization claim the procedure does not treat an illness. The absence of pregnancy, by their definition, is not a disease. In fact, many companies specifically exclude in vitro fertilization as a treatment.

However, the same companies may reimburse for fertility medications and sonograms performed while undergoing in vitro fertilization as legitimate diagnostic procedures. If that is the case, at least part of a couple's expenses may be recouped.

Self-Insured Companies

Companies may fund their own insurance pools under a federal statute called the Employee Retirement Income Security Act of 1974. Many large employers use this method to control health care costs. Although ERISA plans are usually administered by major insurance carriers, self-insured companies design their own coverage. Therefore, reimbursement for in vitro fertilization varies from company to company. Check with the insurance coordinator in your office if you work for a self-insured company.

Insurance Claims

When preparing insurance claims, remember to document, document, document. If a dispute arises about a claim, records make your case stronger. Make copies of every claim submitted and keep them on file for easy reference. To assist you in completing claim forms, write pertinent information in a prominent place where you can locate it.

FINANCIAL POLICIES

Texas Center for Reproductive Health has several policies you should be aware of.

- ❖ **Payment agreement.** At the beginning of your cycle, you will be asked to sign a payment agreement. This agreement states that you will be responsible for paying for all charges by the beginning of stimulation.
- ❖ **Credit card on file.** At the beginning of your treatment, we will request an imprint of a major credit card (Visa, MasterCard, or Discover) and we will use this imprint to process all additional charges exceeding those that were not collected at the time of the beginning of stimulation.
- ❖ **Charges.** You will be given a list of charges that accrue to you during the average IVF/ET cycle. Your charges may be more or less than the average depending on the specifics of your particular case.
- ❖ **Excess funds.** As we collect all costs for your treatment, any payment received by your insurer will be returned to the insurer to be forwarded to you. If monies remain in your account at the conclusion of your treatment, excess funds will be returned to you if you request such a return, or excess funds can remain in your account.

FINANCE OPTIONS

Prosper Healthcare Lending has agreed to finance the costs of an IVF cycle for qualifying applicants. Please ask the receptionist or office manager for information if you are interested.

Acknowledgments

The Center thanks the physicians who have trusted us to care for their patients and the patients who have selected our center to provide procreative care.

This publication would not have been possible without the continued support and work of numerous individuals. Many of these individuals have not worked at the center for years but their support continues. I am certain I will omit some of the individuals who should be listed here, and for such omission, I apologize.

- Dr. Juan Correa-Pérez, laboratory director, andrologist, embryologist—for serving as manuscript author

- Mrs. Sharon Marynick—for her untiring dedication to the work of the Texas Center for Reproductive Health—along with our children, Ashley, Laird, and Mark; our grandchildren, Hannah, Emily, and Rebecca; and our son-in-law, Lee Williams

- Mrs. Susan Owen—for her untiring dedication to the work of the Texas Center for Reproductive Health

- Mr. Galen Johnson, Mr. William S. Carter, and Mr. Boone Powell, Jr., Baylor Health Care System administrators, and Reuben H. Adams, Jr., MD, chief of obstetrics/gynecology at Baylor University Medical Center—for making the center possible in 1983

- Mrs. Betty Sponer, Baylor Health Care System administrator—for being instrumental in the early success of the center

- Mr. Raul Astiazaran-Ybarra, the first full-time embryologist at the center—for checking in yearly to see how our work is going

- Ms. Valerie Rennon—for reviewing the manuscript and her untiring work to produce the final version of this document

- Ms. Jami Lander—for her exceptional dedication to helping our patients and her work as a manuscript reviewer

- Ms. LaKisha Sanders-Massey—for her tireless work helping wherever it is needed

- Mr. Carl Soderstrom, Dr. Merrick Reese, Mr. Larry Friedman, and Mr. Ryan Lurich—for their advice, guidance, and encouragement over a period of years

- Dr. Thomas "Rusty" Pool, Dr. Michael Reed, Dr. Young S. Moon, Dr. Gary Hodgen, Dr. Howard W. Jones, Jr., Dr. Georgeanna Seeger Jones, and Dr. David Meldrum—for sharing their knowledge and allowing us to learn from their experiences over the years

- Dr. Carolyn B. Coulam—for teaching us about the immunology of reproduction and pregnancy
- Dr. Tillmann Hein and Dr. Charles Sessions—for bringing contemporary anesthesiology to the practice of reproductive medicine
- Ms. Ashley Keith—for the completion of the manuscript/manuscript revision
- Mr. Tracy C. Williamson—for technical advice and support
- Mr. Sparky Beckham, Reverend Travis Berry, and Mr. Fred Roach—for encouragement and ethical guidance

Samuel P. Marynick, MD
Dallas, Texas, January 2016

Appendix A:
Outcome Data

The Texas Center for Reproductive Health began performing in vitro fertilization with embryo transfer (IVF/ET) in 1989, the same year the Society for Assisted Reproduction Technology (SART) began collecting treatment outcome data for SART-participating reproduction centers. The graphs depict the total number of IVF/ET cycles performed in SART-participating centers for each year from 1989 to 2013 (Figure 1) and the average pregnancy rates (Figure 2) and delivery rates (Figure 3) for all reporting centers for women under the age of 38 years and for the Texas Center for Reproductive Health over this 24-year period. The Texas Center for Reproductive Health has had consistently better outcomes than the national average.

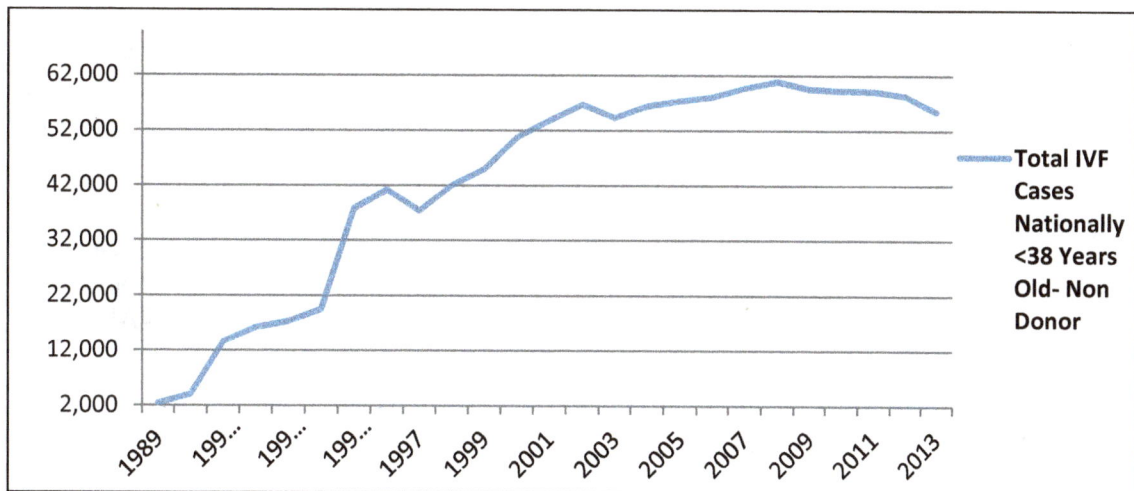

Figure 1. Total IVF cases nationally from 1989 to 2013.

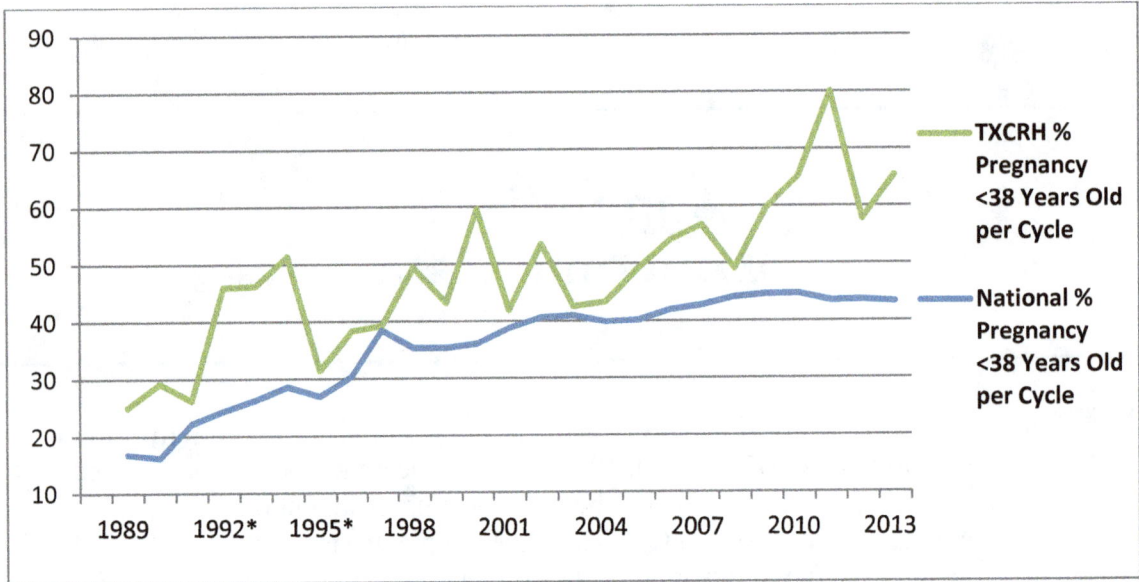

Figure 2. Pregnancy rate from 1989 to 2013 both nationally and for the Texas Center for Reproductive Health.

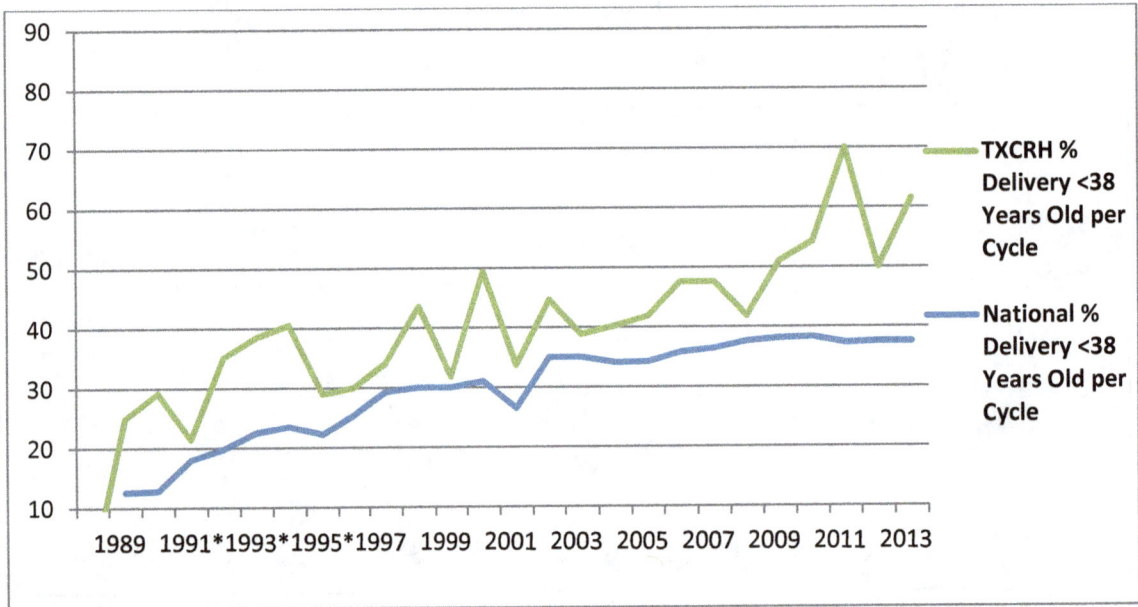

Figure 3. Delivery rate from 1989 to 2013 both nationally and for the Texas Center for Reproductive Health.

Appendix B: Recommended Reading

Websites of Note

1. www.ASRM.org—American Society for Reproductive Medicine
2. www.TXCRH.com—Our website
3. www.Resolve.org—The National Infertility Association
4. www.SART.org—Society for Assisted Reproductive Technology
5. www.CDC.gov—Centers for Disease Control and Prevention
6. www.ESHRE.eu—European Society for Human Reproduction and Embryology

Periodicals

(Available in university and medical libraries)

1. *Fertility and Sterility*—monthly journal
2. *Contemporary OB/GYN*—monthly journal
3. *Obstetrics and Gynecology*—monthly journal
4. *Human Reproduction*—monthly journal
5. *The Journal of Assisted Reproduction and Genetics*—monthly journal

Newsletters

1. *What's New in Fertility?*—published by Resolve, 1310 Broadway, Sommerville, MA 02144-1731 (Available through the national headquarters or local chapters of Resolve or at your local library.)

Books: Learning about Reproduction, Fertility, and Infertility

1. *How To Be a Successful Fertility Patient.* Peggy Robin. William Morrow and Co., Inc., New York, 1993.
2. *Getting Pregnant When You Thought You Couldn't.* Helane S. Rosenbert and Yakov M. Epstein. Grand Central Publishing, New York, 1993.
3. *The Couple's Guide to Fertility.* Gary S. Berger, Marc Goldstein, and Mark Fuerst. Doubleday, New York, 1995.
4. *The American Medical Women's Association Guide to Fertility and Reproductive Health.* Roselyn P. Epps and Susan Cobb Stewart. Dell Publications, New York, 1995.

5. *In Pursuit of Fertility.* Robert R. Franklin and Kay Bockman. Henry Holland Co., New York, 1995.
6. *Taking Charge of Your Fertility. The Definitive Guide to Natural Birth Control and Pregnancy.* Toni Weschler. Harper, New York, 1995.
7. *Dr. Richard Marrs' Fertility Book.* Richard Marrs, MD. Dell, New York, 1997.
8. *Complete Guide to Fertility.* Sandra Ann Carson, MD, and Peter R. Casson, MD. Contemporary Books, Chicago, 1999.
9. *Getting Pregnant.* Niels H. Lanersen, MD, PhD, and Collette Boucher. Simon and Schuster, New York, 2000.
10. *The Infertility Survival Handbook.* Elizabeth Swire-Falker. Riverhead Books, New York, 2004.
11. *Everything Conceivable.* Liza Mundy. Alfred A. Knopf, New York, 2007.
12. *In Vitro Fertilization Comes to America.* Howard W. Jones, Jr., MD. Jamestowne Bookworks, Williamsburg, 2014.

Books: Advanced Reproductive Technologies

1. *Micromanipulation of Human Gametes.* Jacques Cohen. Raven Press, New York, 1992.
2. *New Conceptions: A Consumer's Guide to the Newest Infertility Treatments.* Lori Andrews. St. Martin's Press, New York, 1984.
3. *From Infertility to In-Vitro Fertilization.* Dr. Geoffrey Sher and Virginia Marriage, RN, MN, with Jean Stoess, MA. McGraw-Hill, New York, 1988.
4. *High-Tech Conception.* Brian Kearney, PhD. Bantam Books, New York, 1998.

Books: How It Feels To Be Infertile

1. *Infertility: How Couples Can Cope.* Linda Salazar, MSW. G. K. Hall, Boston, 1986.
2. *Infertility: A Guide for the Childless Couple.* Barbara Eck Menning. Prentice Hall, Englewood Cliffs, NJ, 1977; revised, 1987.
3. *The Miracle Seekers.* Mary Martin Mason. Perspectives Press, Fort Wayne, IN, 1987.
4. *Understanding—A Guide to Impaired Fertility for Family and Friends.* Patricia I. Johnston. Perspectives Press, Fort Wayne, IN, 1983.
5. *Coping with Infertility.* Judith Stigger. Augsberg Publishing, Minneapolis, 1983.
6. *Inconceivable.* Julia Indichova. Broadway Books, New York, 1997. (A wonderful story!)
7. *The Infertility Companion.* Sandra L. Glahn, ThM, and William R. Cutrer, MD. Zondervan, Grand Rapids, 2004.

Books: Miscarriage

1. *Empty Arms: Coping with Miscarriage, Stillbirth, and Infant Death.* Sherokee Ilse. Wintergreen Press, Maple Plains, MN, 1990.
2. *Motherhood after Miscarriage.* Dr. Kathleen Diamond. Bob Adams, Inc., Holbrook, MA, 1991.

3. *Miscarriage. Women Sharing from the Heart.* Marie Allen and Shelly Marks. John Wiley and Sons, New York, 1993.

Books: Legal

1. *Legal Conceptions.* Susan L. Crockin, JD, and Howard W. Jones, Jr., MD. Johns Hopkins University Press, Baltimore, 2010.

Appendix C:
American Society of Reproductive Medicine Fact Sheets

*All fact sheets are from **ReproductiveFacts.org**, the patient education website of the American Society for Reproductive Medicine. Additional fact sheets are available from that site.*

IN VITRO FERTILIZATION: WHAT ARE THE RISKS?

IVF is a method of assisted reproduction in which a man's sperm and a woman's eggs are combined outside of the body in a laboratory dish. One or more fertilized eggs (embryos) may be transferred into the woman's uterus, where they may implant in the uterine lining and develop. Serious complications from IVF medicines and procedures are rare. As with all medical treatments, however, there are some risks. This document discusses the most common risks.

What kind of side effects can occur with IVF medicines?

Usually, injectable fertility medications (gonadotropins) are used for an IVF cycle. These medicines help stimulate a number of follicles with eggs to grow in the ovaries. A more detailed discussion of fertility medications can be found in the ASRM booklet, *Medications for inducing ovulation.*

Possible side effects of injectable fertility medicines include:

- Mild bruising and soreness at the injection site (using different sites for the injections can help)
- Nausea and, occasionally, vomiting
- Temporary allergic reactions, such as skin reddening and/or itching at the injection site
- Breast tenderness and increased vaginal discharge
- Mood swings and fatigue
- Ovarian hyperstimulation syndrome (OHSS)

Most symptoms of OHSS (nausea, bloating, ovarian discomfort) are mild. They usually go away without treatment within a few days after the egg collection. In severe cases, OHSS can cause large amounts of fluid to build up in the abdomen (belly) and lungs. This can cause very enlarged ovaries, dehydration, trouble breathing, and severe abdominal pain.

Very rarely (in less than 1% of women having egg retrieval for IVF), OHSS can lead to blood clots and kidney failure. For more information about OHSS, see the ASRM fact sheet *Ovarian hyperstimulation syndrome (OHSS)*.

Earlier reports from several decades ago suggested a link between ovarian cancer and the use of fertility medicines. However, more recent and well done studies no longer show clear associations between ovarian cancer and the use of fertility medications.

What are the risks of the egg retrieval?

During the egg retrieval, your doctor uses vaginal ultrasound to guide the insertion of a long, thin needle through your vagina into the ovary and then into each follicle to retrieve eggs. Possible risks for this procedure include:

- Mild to moderate pelvic and abdominal pain (during or after). In most cases, the pain disappears within a day or two and can be managed with over-the-counter pain medications.
- Injury to organs near the ovaries, such as the bladder, bowel, or blood vessels. Very rarely, bowel or blood vessel injury can require emergency surgery and, occasionally, blood transfusions.
- Pelvic infection (mild to severe). Pelvic infections following egg retrieval or embryo transfer are now uncommon because antibiotic medicines are usually given at the time of egg collection. Severe infection may require hospitalization and/or treatment with intravenous antibiotics.
- Rarely, to manage a severe infection, surgery may be required to remove one or both of the ovaries and tubes and/or uterus. Women who have had pelvic infections or endometriosis involving the ovaries are more likely to get IVF-related infections.

What are the risks associated with the embryo transfer?

A catheter containing the embryos is used to gently place them into the uterus (womb). Women may feel mild cramping when the catheter is inserted through the cervix or they may have vaginal spotting (slight bleeding) afterward. Very rarely, an infection may develop, which can usually be treated with antibiotics.

If I conceive with IVF, will my pregnancy be more complicated (than if I conceived on my own)?

Having a multiple pregnancy (pregnancy with more than one baby) is more likely with IVF, particularly when more than one embryo is transferred. These pregnancies carry significant risks, including:

- Preterm labor and/or delivery: premature babies (regardless of whether or not they were conceived naturally or with IVF) are at higher risk for health complications such as lung development problems, intestinal infections, cerebral palsy, learning disabilities, language delay, and behavior problems
- Maternal hemorrhage
- Delivery by cesarean section (C-section)
- Pregnancy-related high blood pressure
- Gestational diabetes

The more embryos that are transferred into the uterus, the greater the risk. Your doctor should transfer the minimum number of embryos necessary to provide a high likelihood of pregnancy with the lowest risk of multiple pregnancy. For more information about multiple pregnancy, see the ASRM booklet titled *Multiple pregnancy and birth: twins, triplets and high-order multiples*. One way to avoid multiple pregnancy is to choose to transfer only one embryo at a time. For more information about this, see the ASRM fact sheet *Single embryo transfer.*

Will IVF increase the risk of my child having a birth defect?

The risk of birth defects in the general population is 2%-3%, and is slightly higher among infertile patients. Most of this risk is due to delayed conception and the underlying cause of infertility. Whether or not IVF alone is responsible for birth defects remains under debate and study. However, when intracytoplasmic sperm injection (ICSI) is done along with IVF, there may be an increased risk of birth defects.

In addition, there may be a slight increased risk of sex chromosome (X or Y chromosome) abnormalities with ICSI. However, it is uncertain if these risks are due to the ICSI procedure itself or to problems with the sperm themselves. Men with sperm defects are more likely to have chromosomal abnormalities, which can be transmitted to their children. However, these disorders are extremely rare. Rare genetic syndromes called imprinting disorders may be slightly increased with IVF.

Miscarriage and ectopic pregnancy

The rate of miscarriage after IVF is similar to the rate following natural conception, with the risk going up with the mother's age. The rate of miscarriage may be as low as 15% for women in their 20s to more than 50% for women in their 40s. There is a small risk (1%) of an ectopic (tubal) pregnancy with IVF; however, this rate is similar to women with a history of infertility. If an ectopic pregnancy occurs, a woman may be given medicines to end the pregnancy or surgery to remove it. If you are pregnant and experience a sharp, stabbing pain; vaginal spotting or bleeding; dizziness or fainting; lower back pain; or low blood pressure (from blood loss), and have not had an ultrasound confirming that the pregnancy is in the uterus, call your doctor immediately. These are all signs of a possible ectopic pregnancy. There is a 1% risk for a heterotopic pregnancy after IVF. This is when an embryo implants and grows in the uterus while another embryo implants in the tube, leading to a simultaneous ectopic pregnancy. Heterotopic pregnancies usually require surgery (to remove the ectopic pregnancy). In most cases, the pregnancy in the womb can continue to develop and grow safely after the tubal pregnancy is removed.

Revised 2015

WHAT IS INTRACYTOPLASMIC SPERM INJECTION (ICSI)?

Before a man's sperm can fertilize a woman's egg, the head of the sperm must attach to the outside of the egg. Once attached, the sperm pushes through the outer layer to the inside of the egg (cytoplasm), where fertilization takes place.

Sometimes the sperm cannot penetrate the outer layer, for a variety of reasons. The egg's outer layer may be thick or hard to penetrate or the sperm may be unable to swim. In these cases, a procedure called intracytoplasmic sperm injection (ICSI) can be done along with in vitro fertilization (IVF) to help fertilize the egg. During ICSI, a single sperm is injected directly into the cytoplasm of the egg.

How does ICSI work?

There are two ways that an egg may be fertilized by IVF: traditional and ICSI. In traditional IVF, 50,000 or more swimming sperm are placed next to the egg in a laboratory dish. Fertilization occurs when one of the sperm enters into the cytoplasm of the egg. In the ICSI process, a tiny needle, called a micropipette, is used to inject a single sperm into the center of the egg. With either traditional IVF or ICSI, once fertilization occurs, the fertilized egg (now called an embryo) grows in a laboratory for 1 to 5 days before it is transferred to the woman's uterus (womb).

Why would I need ICSI?

ICSI helps to overcome fertility problems, such as:

- The male partner produces too few sperm to do artificial insemination (intrauterine insemination [IUI]) or IVF.
- The sperm may not move in a normal fashion.
- The sperm may have trouble attaching to the egg.
- A blockage in the male reproductive tract may keep sperm from getting out.
- Eggs have not fertilized by traditional IVF, regardless of the condition of the sperm.
- In vitro matured eggs are being used.
- Previously frozen eggs are being used.

Will ICSI work?

ICSI fertilizes 50% to 80% of eggs. But the following problems may occur during or after the ICSI process:

- Some or all of the eggs may be damaged.
- The egg might not grow into an embryo even after it is injected with sperm.
- The embryo may stop growing.

Once fertilization takes place, a couple's chance of giving birth to a single baby, twins, or triplets is the same if they have IVF with or without ICSI.

Can ICSI affect a baby's development?

If a woman gets pregnant naturally, there is a 1.5% to 3% chance that the baby will have a major birth defect. The chance of birth defects associated with ICSI is similar to IVF, but slightly higher than in natural conception.

The slightly higher risk of birth defects may actually be due to the infertility and not the treatments used to overcome the infertility.

Certain conditions have been associated with the use of ICSI, such as Beckwith-Wiedemann syndrome, Angelman syndrome, hypospadias, or sex chromosome abnormalities. They are thought to occur in far less than 1% of children conceived using this technique.

Some of the problems that cause infertility may be genetic. For example, male children conceived with the use of ICSI may have the same infertility issues as their fathers.

Revised 2014

INFERTILITY COUNSELING AND SUPPORT: WHEN AND WHERE TO FIND IT

Infertility is a medical condition that touches all aspects of your life. It may affect your relationships with others, your perspective on life, and how you feel about yourself. How you deal with these feelings will depend on your personality and life experiences. Most people can benefit from the support of family, friends, medical caregivers, and mental health professionals. When considering infertility treatment options such as sperm, egg, or embryo donation or gestational carriers, it may be especially helpful to gain the assistance of a fertility counselor. The following information may help you decide if you need to seek professional help in managing the emotional stresses associated with fertility treatment or need assistance regarding your treatment options.

When do I need to see an infertility counselor?

Consider counseling if you are feeling depressed, anxious, or so preoccupied with your infertility that you feel it is hard to live your life productively. You also may want to seek the assistance of a counselor if you are feeling "stuck" and need to explore your options. Signs that you might benefit from counseling include:

- Persistent feelings of sadness, guilt, or worthlessness
- Social isolation
- Loss of interest in usual activities and relationships
- Depression
- Agitation and/or anxiety
- Mood swings
- Constant preoccupation with infertility
- Marital problems
- Difficulty with "scheduled" intercourse
- Difficulty concentrating and/or remembering
- Increased use of alcohol or drugs
- A change in appetite, weight, or sleep patterns
- Thoughts about suicide or death

Where can I get support?

Support can come from many different sources. Books can offer information and understanding about the emotional aspects of infertility. Support groups and informational meetings can reduce the feeling of isolation and provide opportunities to learn and share with others experiencing infertility. Individual and couple counseling offer the chance to talk with an experienced professional to sort out your feelings, identify coping mechanisms, and work to find solutions to your difficulties. Discussions with supportive family members and friends also can be useful.

How do I find an infertility counselor or other support?

Start by asking your physician for referrals to trained mental health professionals in your area, a list of relevant books and articles, and support resources that deal with fertility-related matters. Counselors may be psychiatrists, psychologists, social workers, psychiatric nurses, or marriage and family therapists. Visit ReproductiveFacts.org and click on the button labeled "Find a Healthcare Professional" for a list of doctors and mental health professionals in your area.

Are there any specific resources available to guide individuals coping with infertility?

There are many resources included on the ASRM patient website (ReproductiveFacts.org), including frequently asked questions, videos, fact sheets and booklets (many also in Spanish), and ASRM Practice and Ethics statements.

Below are listed several additional resources that may be helpful in addressing a variety of concerns and issues. This list is by no means exhaustive. If you require help regarding other topics, please consult the patient resources section of ReproductiveFacts.org or your healthcare professional.

- American Fertility Association (AFA): An organization created to educate the public about reproductive disease and support families during struggles with infertility and adoption, TheAFA.org
- Choice Moms: An organization to help single women who proactively decide to become the best mother they can, through adoption or conception, choicemoms.org
- Fertile Hope: A national LIVESTRONG initiative dedicated to providing reproductive information, support, and hope to cancer patients and survivors whose medical treatments present the risk of infertility, fertilehope.org
- Frank Talk: A peer-support website dedicated to helping men deal with erectile dysfunction, FrankTalk.org
- International Council on Infertility Information Dissemination, Inc. (INCIID), inciid.org
- North American Council on Adoptable Children: An organization committed to meeting the needs of waiting children and the families who adopt them, nacac.org
- Parents Via Egg Donation: An organization created to provide information to parents and parents-to-be and to share information about all facets of the egg donation process, parentsviaeggdonation.org
- Pop Luck Club: The Pop Luck Club has evolved into a substantial voice, helping to support the growth of our wonderfully diverse LBGT community, popluckclub.org
- RESOLVE: A national infertility support organization, Resolve.org
- Single Mothers by Choice: Offering support and information to single women who are considering motherhood and to single mothers who have chosen this path to parenthood, singlemothersbychoice.org
- Magazines: *Fertility Road, Fertility Magazine, Conceive Magazine, Gay Parent Magazine*

Revised 2014

Appendix D:
Contacts

RESOLVE
National Headquarters
1310 Broadway
Sommerville, MA 02144-1731
(617) 623-1156; Fax: (617) 623-0252; Helpline: (617) 623-0744
E-mail: resolveinc@aol.com
Dallas/Fort Worth Chapter: (214) 621-7560

THE ENDOMETRIOSIS ASSOCIATION
PO Box 92187
Milwaukee, WI 53202
(414) 355-2200
1-800-992-3636

PREGNANCY AND INFANT LOSS CENTER
1415 E. Wayzata Blvd., Suite 22
Wayzata, MN 55391
(612) 473-9372

THE AMERICAN SOCIETY FOR REPRODUCTIVE MEDICINE
Formerly The American Fertility Society
1209 Montgomery Highway
Birmingham, AL 35216-2809
(205) 978-5000
Fax: (205) 975-5005
E-mail: asrm@asrm.com

ADOPTIVE FAMILIES OF AMERICA
33 Highway 100 N.
Minneapolis, MN 55422
(800) 372-3300

NORTH AMERICAN COINCIL ON ADOPTIVE CHILDREN
1821 University Avenue #498 N.
St. Paul, MN 55104
(612) 644-0336

Appendix E: Glossary

American Society of Reproductive Medicine: A professional society of physicians, laboratory personnel, psychologists, nurses, and other paramedical personnel interested in fertility and disorders of fertility.

Augmented laparoscopy: A procedure in which eggs are retrieved from the woman's ovaries while a diagnostic laparoscopy is performed to evaluate the integrity of her pelvic organs. Eggs are later fertilized in a laboratory and pre-embryos are transferred into the woman's uterus several days later.

Basal body temperature chart: A daily body temperature chart that provides a rough idea of when ovulation occurred. This is possible because body temperature rises just after ovulation when the corpus luteum produces progesterone and drops at or just before the beginning of menstruation, when estrogen and progesterone levels fall.

Bravelle®: *see* follicle-stimulating hormone.

Capacitation: The process that occurs in sperm as they pass through the woman's reproductive tract that allows sperm to fertilize eggs. This same sperm maturation can occur in the laboratory when sperm are maintained in an incubator.

Cellular cleavage: The process of cell division.

Cervical canal: The connection between the outer cervical opening and the uterine cavity.

Cervical mucus: Mucus produced by glands in the cervical canal. This mucus plays an important role in selecting out only the best sperm for movement into the uterus and initiates the sperm capacitation process.

Cervical mucus insufficiency: A condition where the ability of the cervical mucus to initiate the capacitation process is compromised or where the mucus does not allow for sperm penetration into the uterus. Causes include production of an insufficient amount of mucus, abnormality in the physical-chemical makeup of the mucus produced caused by the presence of infection in the glands of the cervix, an abnormal hormonal environment, or the secretion of antibodies to sperm in the mucus. Cervical mucus abnormalities are responsible for about 10% of all cases of infertility.

Cervix: Lowermost part of the uterus. Extends into the upper vagina and opens into the uterus through the narrow endocervical canal.

Chemical pregnancy: Biochemical evidence of a possible developing pregnancy based on a positive blood or urine pregnancy test; at this point, pregnancy is presumptive until confirmed by ultrasound.

Chlamydia: A bacterial sexually transmitted infection. The bacterium may damage fallopian tubes and/or male reproductive tracts, thereby causing infertility.

Clinical pregnancy: A pregnancy that has been confirmed by ultrasound examination or through pathologic examination of a surgical specimen obtained either from a miscarriage or from an ectopic pregnancy.

Conception: Creation of a zygote by the fertilization of an egg.

Conceptus: A term used to describe the developing implanted embryo and/or early fetus.

Controlled ovarian hyperstimulation: Response of the ovary to the administration of fertility medication with the maturation of several follicles simultaneously. This generally results in the production of multiple ova by these follicles with an exaggerated hormonal response compared to the natural menstrual cycle.

Corpus luteum: A term for a follicle after an egg has been released. After ovulation, the follicle collapses, turns yellow, and is transformed biochemically and hormonally into the corpus luteum. The corpus luteum produces progesterone and estrogen and has a life span of about 10 to 14 days, after which it atrophies unless a pregnancy occurs. If the woman becomes pregnant, the life span of the corpus luteum is prolonged for many weeks.

Cryopreservation: The process of freezing in liquid nitrogen and storing eggs, sperm, and pre-embryos for future use.

Cul-de-sac: Area of the woman's abdominal cavity behind the lower part of the uterus.

Cumulus mass: A mass of cells that surround the human egg; the corona radiata are those cumulus cells that are closest to the egg and resemble a sunburst.

E2: *see* estradiol.

Ectopic pregnancy: A pregnancy that occurs when the embryo attempts to implant in a location other than the uterus, most commonly the fallopian tube. If undetected, an ectopic pregnancy may rupture and cause life-threatening internal bleeding; ectopic pregnancies frequently require surgical intervention. Early ectopic pregnancies may be treated in many cases using the chemotherapy medication methotrexate.

Egg: The female gamete, which develops in the ovary; also known as an ovum or oocyte. An egg is the largest cell in the body.

Egg retrieval: Retrieval of eggs from ovarian follicles prior to ovulation. Eggs are aspirated out of the follicles through a needle either during laparoscopy or under vaginal ultrasound guidance.

Embryo: Term for a fertilized egg from the time it first develops a primitive streak (about 2 weeks after fertilization) through the first 6 to 8 weeks of gestation.

Embryo transfer: Transferring pre-embryos that were started in vitro to the uterus.

Endometrial biopsy: Surgical removal of a specimen of the endometrium to microscopically examine the effect of estrogen and progesterone on the endometrium. This is generally performed using a 1.5 mm flexible plastic device called a Pipell™.

Endometriosis: A condition in which endometrial-like tissue grows outside the uterus, which may cause scarring, pain, and bleeding, often damaging the fallopian tubes and ovaries in the process.

Endometrium: The lining of the uterus which grows during the menstrual cycle under the influence of estrogen and progesterone. The endometrium grows in anticipation of nurturing an implanting embryo in the event of a pregnancy. It sloughs off in the form of menstruation if pre-embryo implantation does not occur.

Estradiol (E2): A female hormone produced by ovarian follicles. The concentration of estrogen in the woman's blood is often measured to determine the degree of her response to controlled ovarian hyperstimulation with fertility medication and to assess the maturity of ovarian follicles.

Estrogen: A primary female sex hormone produced by the ovaries, the placenta, and to a small degree by the adrenal gland.

Fallopian tubes: Narrow 4-inch long hollow structures that lead from the sides of the uterus to the ovaries.

Fertility medications: Natural or synthetic compounds that are administered to a woman in order to stimulate her ovaries to produce more mature eggs than usual or administered to a man in an attempt to enhance sperm number and function.

Fertilization: The fusion of the sperm and egg to form a zygote.

Flare protocol: The use of gonadotropin-releasing hormone agonists/antagonists in very small dosages to stimulate the pituitary gland to release luteinizing hormone and follicle-stimulating hormone to aid in the stimulation of the ovary to form follicles.

Follicle-stimulating hormone (FSH): A gonadotropin that is released by the pituitary gland to stimulate the ovaries or testicles. This comes as a medication that may be given intramuscularly or subcutaneously. Bravelle®, Gonal-F®, Follistim®, and several other brand-name preparations are medications utilized in ovarian stimulation that are composed of follicle-stimulating hormone.

Follicles: Cyst-like structures within the ovary that produce the female hormones estrogen and progesterone and produce the female gamete or egg.

Follistim®: *see* follicle-stimulating hormone.

Fornix: Deep recesses in the upper vagina created by the protrusion of the cervix into the roof of the vagina.

Gamete: Female egg and male sperm.

Gamete intrafallopian transfer (GIFT): A therapeutic gamete-related technique that involves the placement of one or more eggs with washed, capacitated, and incubated sperm directly into the fallopian tubes so that fertilization can occur at the location of natural gamete fertilization.

Gonadotropin-releasing hormone (GnRH): A messenger hormone released by the hypothalamus to influence the production and release of gonadotropins (luteinizing hormone, follicle-stimulating hormone) by the pituitary gland.

Gonadotropin-releasing hormone agonists/antagonists: GnRH-like hormones that stimulate or block the body's release of both follicle-stimulating hormone and luteinizing hormone. By blocking luteinizing hormone production, GnRH agonists improve the predictability of a woman's response to fertility medication.

Gonadotropins: Luteinizing hormone and follicle-stimulating hormone which are released from the pituitary gland to initiate the reproductive process by stimulating testicles and ovaries.

Gonal-F®: *see* follicle-stimulating hormone.

Growth medium: A solution that promotes cleavage and development of a pre-embryo.

Hormonal insufficiency: In IVF, hormonal insufficiency may be caused by an abnormal response to fertility medication and may lead to the failure of an embryo to implant because the amount of hormones produced and the timing of their production and release are not synchronized.

Hormone: A substance made in one place in the body which moves through the body to produce an effect in another part of the body.

Human chorionic gonadotropin (hCG): A hormone produced by the implanting placenta which indicates a possible pregnancy. Injections of hCG may be given following embryo transfer to encourage production of progesterone by the corpus luteum to promote implantation and thereby reduce the risk of spontaneous miscarriage. hCG produced by the placenta in an early pregnancy is what normally maintains the corpus luteum produced as a part of ovulation. It is the progesterone produced by the corpus luteum hormone under the influence of hCG that allows the uterus to accept a heterograft (non-self) implantation. The hCG that is used for injection is derived from the urine of pregnant women.

Human menopausal gonadotropin (hMG): A medication made from the urine of menopausal women that contains luteinizing hormone and follicle-stimulating hormone. Menopur® is a brand name preparation of hMG.

Hypothalamus: A small area in the mid-portion of the brain that works with the pituitary gland to regulate the formation and release of pituitary hormones.

Implantation: The process that occurs when the pre-embryo burrows into the endometrium and eventually connects to the mother's circulatory system.

In vitro fertilization (IVF): Literally meaning fertilization in glass, IVF comprises several steps: stimulation of ovaries with fertility medication, retrieval of eggs by suction through a needle, fertilization of eggs with sperm, and subsequent pre-embryo transfer to the uterus.

Infertility: The inability to conceive after one full year of normal heterosexual intercourse without the use of contraception.

Intracytoplasmic sperm injection (ICSI): The placement of a sperm using micromanipulation inside the egg cytoplasm to seek to enhance the likelihood of egg fertilization.

Laparoscope: A long, thin telescope-like instrument containing a high intensity light source and a system of lenses that enables the physician to examine the abdominal cavity and to perform other diagnostic or surgical procedures under direct vision without necessitating major surgery.

Laparoscopy: A surgical procedure using the laparoscope. Laparoscopy may be used for egg retrieval, diagnostic evaluation, reparative surgery, and various other fertility procedures. (This may be performed as micro laparoscopy in some cases, which requires less anesthesia.)

Lithotomy: Position that a woman is asked to assume in order to undergo a gynecological examination or other procedures such as embryo transfer and vaginal ultrasound examination.

Lupron®: A commonly used GnRH agonist/antagonist. *See* gonadotropin-releasing hormone agonists/antagonists.

Luteinizing hormone (LH): A gonadotropin released by the pituitary gland to stimulate the ovaries and testicles. It is the hormone released just prior to ovulation that produces the final egg maturation steps.

Menopur®: *see* human menopausal gonadotropin.

Menstrual cycle: The time that elapses between menstrual periods. An average cycle is 28 days. Ovulation occurs at the midpoint, around the 14th day.

Micromanipulation: The use of very fine glass tools to manipulate eggs and sperm to enhance egg fertilization or in pre-embryos to enhance implantation of pre-embryos in the uterus.

Micro-organelles: Tiny intracellular factories that produce energy and perform metabolic functions in the egg, pre-embryos, and other cells.

Miscarriage: Spontaneous expulsion of the products of conception from the uterus during the first half of pregnancy.

Motility: The ability of sperm to move and progress forward through the reproductive tract and to fertilize the egg.

Multiple pregnancy: The presence of more than one embryo implanted within the woman's uterus.

Nucleus: Structure in the cell that bears genetic material.

Oocyte: *see* egg.

Ooplasm: Nurturing material around the nucleus of the egg that contains micro-organelles and nurtures the zygote and pre-embryo after fertilization.

Ovaries: Two white, almond-like structures (the female counterpart of the testicles) that are attached to either side of the pelvis adjacent to the ends of the fallopian tubes. The ovaries release eggs, secrete sex hormones, and secrete peptide hormones into the bloodstream.

Ovulation: When an ovary releases one or more eggs.

Ovum: *see* egg.

Patency: Openness, freedom from blockage, particularly referring to the fallopian tubes.

Percoll™: A molecular filter used to separate sperm from seminal plasma and other constituents of the semen such as bacteria and white blood cells. Isolate™ has replaced Percoll™ in ART procedures.

Pituitary gland: An organ the size of a small grape that sits at the base of the brain and interacts with the hypothalamus to regulate and release many hormones in the body.

Placenta: The organ formed in the lining of the uterus by the uterine mucous membranes with the membranes of the fetus to provide for the nourishment of the fetus and the elimination of fetal waste products.

Polyspermia: Entrance of more than one sperm into an egg during fertilization. This causes the zygote to die or the embryo to divide haphazardly and then die, as the conception has an abnormal number of chromosomes.

Pre-embryo: The term for a fertilized egg from sperm penetration and nuclear fusion until a primitive streak (earliest evidence of a new unique human being) is formed about 14 days after fertilization.

Progesterone: A primary female sex hormone produced by the corpus luteum that induces secretory changes in the glands of the endometrium. Progesterone may also be given by injection, orally, or in the form of vaginal gels or suppositories to enhance implantation and to seek to reduce the risk of miscarriage. Progesterone is made by the placenta in the latter part of the first trimester and in the second and third trimesters of pregnancy.

Semen: The combination of sperm, seminal fluid, and other male reproductive secretions.

Semen analysis: A basic fertility assessment test of sperm function, primarily involving counting the number of sperm, assessing their motility and progression, and evaluating sperm overall structure and form.

Sperm: Male gamete or spermatozoa.

Subzonal sperm insertion (SUZI): The placement of several sperm under the eggshell (zona pellucida) using micromanipulation to seek to enhance the likelihood of egg fertilization, generally no longer utilized as ICSI produces more predictable fertilization results than SUZI.

Superovulation: Ovulation of more than one egg induced by the administration of fertility medication.

Testicles: The male counterparts of the female ovaries; located in the scrotum, the testicles produce sperm and male hormones such as testosterone.

Testosterone: The predominant male sex hormone which influences the production and maturation of sperm.

Transvaginal egg retrieval: An ultrasound-guided egg retrieval procedure in which the retrieving needle is passed through the top of the woman's vagina into her ovaries under ultrasound guidance.

Treatment cycle: The menstrual cycle during which a particular fertility treatment such as IVF is or was performed.

Ultrasound: A painless diagnostic procedure that transforms high-frequency sound waves as they travel through body tissue and fluid into images on a monitor. It enables the physician to clearly identify structures within the body and to guide instruments during procedures. Ultrasound is also used to diagnose and follow the progress of a clinical pregnancy.

Unexplained infertility: Infertility whose cause cannot readily be determined by conventional diagnostic procedures; this occurs in about 10% of all infertile couples.

Urine ovulation tests (urinary LH testing): A simple test that can pinpoint the time of presumed ovulation. Regular charting of the test results detects the surge of luteinizing hormone that triggers ovulation and precedes ovulation by about 24 hours. Urinary luteinizing hormone testing is generally performed on the second voided urine sample of the day.

Uterus: A muscular organ that enlarges during pregnancy from its normal pear size to accommodate a full-term pregnancy.

Vagina: The passage that leads from the vulva to the cervix. The vagina's elastic tissues have remarkable ability to stretch.

Washing: Processing of a semen specimen using a centrifuge in order to separate the sperm from seminal plasma. The sperm are then resuspended in media and separated again by centrifugation.

Zona-cumulus complex: Mass of cells through which the sperm must pass to reach the egg.

Zona hatching: The opening of the zona pellucida (eggshell) using micromanipulation to seek to enhance the likelihood of pre-embryo implantation in the uterus.

Zona pellucida: The shell-like covering of the human egg.

Zona splitting (or drilling): The opening of the zona pellucida (eggshell) using micromanipulation to seek to enhance the likelihood of egg fertilization (not utilized much at the present time).

Zygote: Term for a fertilized egg until it begins to cleave, at which time it is known as a pre-embryo.

Source: Modified from *Infertility to In-Vitro Fertilization,* by Dr. Geoffrey Sher and Virginia Marriage, RN, MN, with Jean Stoess, MA.

NOTES